Red light
Therapy

Learn step-by-step how to use red light treatment
for fat loss, anti-aging, muscle gain, fatigue and pain.

Table of Contents

Introduction

Red light treatment (RLT) is a disputable helpful strategy that utilizations red low-level wavelengths of light to treat skin issues, for example, wrinkles, scars, and diligent injuries, among different conditions.

In the mid 1990s, RLT was utilized by researchers to help develop plants in space. The researchers found that the exceptional light from red light-discharging diodes (LEDs) advanced development and photosynthesis of plant cells.

Red light was then read for its potential application in medication, all the more explicitly to see whether RLT could expand vitality inside human cells. The specialists trusted that RLT could be a viable method to treat the muscle decay, slow twisted recuperating, and bone thickness issues brought about by weightlessness during space travel.

You may have known about red light treatment (RLT) by its different names, which include:

- photobiomodulation (PBM)
- low level light treatment (LLLT)

- delicate laser treatment
- cold laser treatment
- biostimulation
- photonic incitement
- low-control laser treatment (LPLT)

When RLT is utilized with photosensitizing meds, it's alluded to as photodynamic treatment. In this sort of treatment, the light just fills in as an enacting operator for the prescription.

There are a wide range of kinds of red light treatment. Red light beds found at salons are said to help lessen corrective skin issues, similar to extend checks and wrinkles. Red light treatment utilized in a restorative office setting might be utilized to treat progressively genuine conditions, similar to psoriasis, slow-mending wounds, and even the symptoms of chemotherapy.

While there's a decent measure of proof to show that RLT might be a promising treatment for specific conditions, there's still a long way to go about how it functions, as well.

How does red light treatment work?

Red light is thought to work by delivering a biochemical

impact in cells that fortifies the mitochondria. The mitochondria are the powerhouse of the cell — it's the place the cell's vitality is made. The vitality conveying atom found in the phones of every single living thing is called ATP (adenosine triphosphate).

By expanding the capacity of the mitochondria utilizing RLT, a cell can make more ATP. With more vitality, cells can work all the more productively, restore themselves, and fix harm.

RLT is not the same as laser or exceptional beat light (IPL) treatments since it doesn't make harm the skin surface. Laser and beat light treatments work by making controlled harm the external layer of the skin, which at that point prompts tissue fix. RLT sidesteps this cruel advance by straightforwardly animating recovery of the skin. The light discharged by RLT enters about 5 millimeters underneath the skin's surface.

How is red light treatment utilized?

As far back as the underlying trials in space, there have been several clinical investigations and a huge number of research facility ponders directed to decide whether RLT has health advantages.

Numerous investigations have had promising outcomes, yet the advantages of red light treatment are as yet a wellspring of discussion. The Centers for Medicare and Medicaid Services (CMS), for instance, has confirmed that there isn't sufficient proof to show that these gadgets are superior to at present existing medications for treating wounds, ulcers, and agony.

Extra clinical research is expected to demonstrate that RLT is compelling. Right now, nonetheless, there's some proof to propose that RLT may have the accompanying advantages:

- advances wound mending and tissue fix
- improves hair development in individuals with androgenic alopecia
- help for the transient treatment of carpal passage disorder
- animates mending of moderate recuperating wounds, similar to diabetic foot ulcers
- diminishes psoriasis injuries
- helps with transient alleviation of torment and morning solidness in individuals with rheumatoid joint pain
- lessens a portion of the symptoms of disease medicines, including oral mucositisTrusted

Source

- improves skin composition and constructs collagenTrusted Source to lessen wrinkles
- repairs sun
- keeps repeating mouth blisters from herpes simplex infection diseases
- improves the soundness of joints in individuals with degenerative osteoarthritis of the knee
- decreases scars
- mitigates torment and inflammationTrusted Source in individuals with torment in the Achilles ligaments

As of now, RLT isn't supported or secured by insurance agencies for these conditions because of absence of adequate proof. Albeit, a couple of insurance agencies presently spread the utilization of RLT to counteract oral mucositis during malignant growth treatment.

Be that as it may, does red light treatment truly work?

While the web is frequently buzzing with news about marvel medications for pretty much every wellbeing condition, red light treatment surely isn't a fix just for everything. RLT is viewed as trial for most conditions.

There's constrained to-no proof indicating that red light treatment does the accompanying:

- treats sadness, regular full of feeling issue, and post birth anxiety
- initiates the lymphatic framework to help "detoxify" the body
- supports the invulnerable framework
- lessens cellulite
- helps in weight reduction
- treats back or neck torment
- battles periodontitis and dental contaminations
- fixes skin inflammation
- treats malignancy

Note that when RLT is utilized with malignancy medicines, the light is just used to initiate another prescription. Other light treatments have been utilized to help with a portion of the conditions above. For example, thinks about have discovered that white light treatment is more successful at treating side effects of misery than red light. Blue light treatment is all the more generally utilized for skin inflammation, with constrained viability.

Are there comparable treatment alternatives?

Red light wavelengths aren't the main wavelengths to be read for restorative purposes. Blue light, green light, and a blend of various wavelengths have additionally been the subject of comparable trials in people.

There are different sorts of light-based treatments accessible. You can get some information about:

- laser medications
- regular daylight
- blue or green light treatment
- sauna light treatment
- bright light B (UVB)
- psoralen and bright light A (PUVA)

Picking a supplier

Many tanning salons, rec centers, and nearby day spas offer RLT for corrective applications. You can likewise discover FDA-endorsed gadgets online that you can buy and use at home. Costs will change. You can have a go at utilizing these gadgets to battle the indications of maturing, similar to age spots, scarcely discernible differences, and wrinkles, however make a point to peruse the directions cautiously. Look at certain gadgets on the web.

For more focused on RLT, you'll have to see a dermatologist first. You may require a few medicines before you notice any distinction.

To treat genuine ailments, similar to malignancy, joint pain, and psoriasis, you should make a meeting with your primary care physician to talk about your alternatives.

Symptoms

Red light treatment is viewed as protected and easy. Nonetheless, there have been reports of consumes and rankling from utilizing RLT units. A couple of individuals created consumes in the wake of nodding off with the unit set up, while others encountered consumes because of broken wires or gadget erosion.

There's additionally a potential danger of harm to the eyes. Albeit more secure on the eyes than conventional lasers, appropriate eye assurance ought to consistently be utilized while experiencing red light treatment.

Takeaway

RLT has indicated promising outcomes in treating some skin conditions, however inside established researchers, there's very little agreement about the treatment's advantages. In light of the momentum inquire about, you may find that RLT is a decent device to add to your healthy skin routine. Continuously check with your PCP or dermatologist before taking a stab at something new.

You can without much of a stretch buy red light gadgets on the web, however it's ideal to hear a specialist's point of view on any indications before you attempt to self-treat. Remember that RLT isn't FDA-endorsed for most conditions or secured by insurance agencies. Any genuine condition, similar to psoriasis, joint inflammation, slow-mending wounds, or agony ought to be looked at by a specialist.

There is some proof to back up a considerable lot of these cases, however RLT is no supernatural occurrence fix.

Anybody considering the treatment ought to likewise find a way to advance skin wellbeing. Inappropriate utilization of RLT may likewise cause some reactions.

Any individual who is unsure about whether RLT is directly for them should converse with their primary care physician.

How it functions

RLT is a clear technique including presenting the body to low wavelength red light. Low-level laser light treatment is another name for the procedure, however RLT might be increasingly normal.

This red light is normal and can infiltrate profound into the skin, where the cells can ingest and utilize it.

As an investigation in the diary Seminars in Cutaneous Medicine and SurgeryTrusted Source notes, mitochondria in the skin cells can ingest these light particles. This can enable the cells to deliver more adenosine triphosphate, which is the vitality hotspot for all cells.

Numerous specialists property the potential positive advantages of RLT to this capacity. With this additional vitality, the cells might have the option to react better to harm and revive themselves.

Despite the fact that there is early research

encompassing RLT, there is still no decisive proof that it is a valuable treatment. Numerous investigations show that the treatment has guarantee, yet progressively broad clinical examinations in people will help decide the potential uses of RLT.

All things considered, there are a few potential advantages of RLT, which we will cover in the segments beneath.

Improving skin wellbeing

The vast majority show enthusiasm for RLT as a potential method to improve skin wellbeing.

The potential for utilizing RLT as an approach to revive the skin has prompted an enormous number of studies. As the survey in the diary Seminars in Cutaneous Medicine and SurgeryTrusted Source notes, RLT may help revive the skin by:

- expanding collagen generation in the skin, which gives the skin its flexibility
- expanding fibroblast generation, which helps produce collagen and other tissue filaments
- expanding course among blood and tissue cells
- shielding cells from harm

- expanding mRNA in the cells, which invigorates the cell
- improving facial surface
- diminishing scarcely discernible differences
- diminishing wrinkle seriousness

A clinical preliminary in the diary Photomedicine and Laser SurgeryTrusted Sourceexplored light treatment for some fundamental skin issues in a little gathering of 136 individuals. The analysts found that these light treatments could:

- restore the skin
- improve the appearance
- improve the sentiment of the skin

It is essential to recollect that a large number of the outcomes with respect to RLT originate from creature or test tube ponders, which investigate the capacity of RLT. A considerable lot of the human investigations utilized little example sizes, as is obvious in the clinical preliminary above.

These outcomes show the potential for the treatment yet are not decisive proof that it will work for each situation.

Improving skin inflammation

RLT may be a viable treatment for skin inflammation vulgaris.

As the survey in Seminars in Cutaneous Medicine and SurgeryTrusted Source additionally notes, types of light treatment are potential options for the treatment of skin break out vulgaris.

Daylight can change the manner in which the sebaceous organs carry on. The sebaceous organs produce sebum, which may stop up the pores and cause skin break out. Daylight may help quiet overactive organs.

The issue that numerous individuals have with daylight presentation is that it accompanies introduction to ultraviolent (UV) An and UVB beams, which may cause other skin issues after some time. These can be serious and may incorporate creating skin disease.

RLT, either alone or in blend with different medications, for example, blue light treatment, is a conceivably powerful treatment for skin break out vulgaris. The light seems to infiltrate profound into the skin and influence sebum generation while additionally lessening aggravation and bothering in the territory.

Wound mending

Red light may likewise be useful in accelerating wound mending.

Research in the diary Anais Brasileiros de DermatologiaTrusted Source features the way that light treatment may help twisted recuperating in a couple of ways, for example, by:

- decreasing irritation in the cells
- invigorating fresh recruits vessels to frame, which specialists call angiogenesis
- expanding supportive fibroblasts in the skin
- expanding collagen creation in the skin
- More examinations in people can help affirm these outcomes.

Expect top to bottom, science-sponsored toplines of our best stories consistently. Tap in and keep your interest fulfilled.

Hair development

A little report in the Journal of Cosmetic and Laser Therapy investigated the impact of low-level light on individuals with alopecia.

The examination uncovered that individuals who got RLT had improved hair thickness, contrasted and those in a control gathering.

The creators note that the impact was gainful when individuals applied light in wavelengths of both 665 nanometres (nm) and 808 nm.

Be that as it may, this was a littler report, and progressively broad clinical investigations will help offer sponsorship to these cases.

Decreasing torment

RLT may likewise be a viable treatment for torment in individuals with specific conditions.

An audit in the European Journal of Physical and Rehabilitation Medicine aggregated the aftereffects of numerous examinations encompassing RLT and musculoskeletal issue.

The exploration showed that RLT could adequately lessen torment in grown-ups with various musculoskeletal issue. The analysts note that professionals who adhere to the particular dose suggestions appear to build the adequacy of the treatment.

Improving bone recuperation

A survey in the Journal of Photochemistry and PhotobiologyTrusted Source analyzes the potential for RLT in treating facial bone imperfections.

The specialists' outcomes demonstrate that RLT may help quicken recuperating after treatment for facial bone deformities. The audit additionally takes note of that the treatment decreased irritation and agony during the procedure.

Be that as it may, the analysts called for an increasingly institutionalized way to deal with decide if the treatment is successful.

Mitigating benefits

As research in the diary AIMS BiophysicsTrusted Source notes, a large number of the conditions that RLT treats have their foundations in aggravation.

In spite of the fact that the careful explanation isn't yet

clear, RLT has huge calming impacts in the body. These impacts are both neighborhood, where experts apply the light, and foundational, in different tissues and organs in the body.

The scientists clarify that the accommodating calming impacts of RLT, and the potential uses for this treatment, are rich.

Further research may assist us with comprehension on the off chance that it might help with interminable fiery issues, for example,

Alzheimer's ailment

- heftiness
- type 2 diabetes
- alopecia areata
- immune system thyroiditis, or irritation of the thyroid
- psoriasis
- joint inflammation
- tendinitis, or irritation of the ligaments

Once more, the examination is as yet primer. Be that as it may, the mitigating impact of RLT is promising.

Past examinations have focused on the significance of the particular wavelengths that individuals use to focus on their skin.

Nonetheless, as the audit in Seminars in Cutaneous Medicine and SurgeryTrusted Source clarifies, the gathered research found that much of the time, the quite certain wavelengths had moderately little effect during treatment.

All things considered, the recurrence for most RLT sessions will commonly differ inside a range, like the wavelengths in the Journal of Photochemistry and PhotobiologyTrusted Source paper.

Potential reactions

RLT is a totally normal procedure. It opens the skin to levels of light that are not hurtful — dissimilar to UV light originating from the sun.

Along these lines, there is for all intents and purposes no danger of symptoms from experiencing RLT. Be that as it may, an expert with little experience or somebody who opens themselves to a lot of the treatment may cause tissue and cell harm.

Items for use at home may likewise prompt abuse, making harm the skin, consumes, or harm to unprotected eyes.

Expenses and protection inclusion

RLT is accessible in various exercise centers, day spas, and tanning salons.

RLT has a generally low working expense. It is likewise not a prescription in the customary sense, so it is broadly accessible. Numerous foundations may offer RLT rooms or lights, including:

- exercise centers
- day spas
- tanning salons
- wellbeing focuses
- saunas
- dermatology workplaces

Numerous organizations additionally offer items that utilization focused on red light lights as a spot mending device. Anybody obtaining such gadgets for use at home should check to be certain that the gadget conveys red light inside the powerful wavelengths before finishing the buy.

There is no protection inclusion for the general act of RLT. In any case, a few dermatologists may offer focused on RLT applications. Any individual who has concerns with respect to a skin issue that RLT may help should see their primary care physician for a referral.

Red light treatment (RLT) is a treatment that may help skin, muscle tissue, and different pieces of your body mend. It opens you to low degrees of red or close infrared light. Infrared light is a sort of vitality your eyes can't see, yet your body can feel as warmth. Red light is like infrared, yet you can see it.

Red light treatment is likewise called low-level laser treatment (LLLT), low-control laser treatment (LPLT), and photobiomodulation (PBM).

How Does Red Light Therapy Work?

With red light treatment, you open your skin to a light, gadget, or laser with a red light. A piece of your phones called mitochondria, at times called the "control generators" of your phones, absorb it and make more vitality. A few specialists think this assists cells with fixing themselves and become more advantageous. This spikes recuperating in skin and muscle tissue.

Things You're Not Telling Your Doctor

Indeed, even the most wellbeing cognizant among us may not tell our PCPs every bit of relevant information when we see them.

Simplicity Secondary Progressive MS With Lifestyle Changes

Medication isn't the best way to treat optional dynamic different sclerosis (SPMS). Diet, work out, and different changes to your day by day schedule could likewise help decrease your side effects.

7 Things to Keep Clean During Cold and Flu Season

Germs that reason colds and influenza can live pretty much anyplace, particularly puts that you don't think to clean frequently. Here are seven hotspots to sanitize.

Red light treatment utilizes extremely low degrees of warmth and doesn't damage or consume the skin. It's not a similar kind of light utilized in tanning corners, and it doesn't open your skin to harming UV beams.

What Does It Treat?

Analysts have thought about red light treatment for some time. Be that as it may, there aren't a great deal of concentrates on it, and they don't have the foggiest idea whether it's superior to anything different kinds of treatment used to enable you to mend. Red light treatment may help with:

Dementia. In one little investigation, individuals with dementia who got ordinary close infrared light treatment on their heads and through their noses for 12 weeks would be wise to recollections, dozed better, and were furious less frequently.

Dental torment. In another little investigation, individuals with temporomandibular brokenness disorder (TMD) had less torment, clicking, and jaw delicacy after red light treatment.

Male pattern baldness. One examination found that people with androgenetic alopecia (a hereditary issue that causes balding) who utilized an at-home RLT gadget for 24 weeks developed thicker hair. Individuals in the investigation who utilized a phony RLT gadget didn't get similar outcomes.

Osteoarthritis. One investigation discovered red and infrared light treatment cut osteoarthritis-related agony by over half.

Tendinitis. A little investigation of 7 individuals recommends RLT diminishes aggravation and torment in individuals with Achilles tendinitis.

Wrinkles and different indications of skin maturing and skin harm. Research shows RLT may smooth your skin and help with wrinkles. RLT likewise assists with skin inflammation scars, consumes, and indications of UV sun harm.

What is red light treatment and what would it be able to treat?

Red light treatment is a remedial procedure that utilizations red, low-level wavelengths of light. At the point when presented to red light treatment, the body creates a biochemical impact that lifts the measure of vitality put away in cells, clarifies Z. Paul Lorenc, M.D., a board-confirmed plastic specialist. This causes cells to work all the more proficiently and fix harm, which is the reason it's been utilized to treat scars and wounds. Be that as it may, red light treatment truly took off in ubiquity for its adequacy in fighting wrinkles, scarcely discernible differences, sun spots, staining, and different indications of not exactly outstanding skin wellbeing.

"Your appearance will be progressively lifted, conditioned, and improved-bringing about more youthful looking, smoother skin by expanding solid cell action," says Vargas. Notwithstanding hydrating and mend the skin, it's likewise incredible for hostile to maturing in light of the fact that it secures existing collagen and elastin, while additionally invigorating new collagen generation, she says. (Related: Are Collagen Supplements Worth It?)

Dr. Lorenc backs up its enemy of maturing powers: "I've worked widely with red light treatment and the skin and see it as compelling at both boosting collagen generation and lessening the presence of barely recognizable differences and wrinkles," he says.

What's more, since the wavelengths infiltrate profoundly, they're more strong than state, a wrinkle-decreasing serum. Utilize the two couple, however, and you'll get results that are (informally) twice as decent.

Would red be able to light help with recuperation?

Red light treatment can likewise treat aggravation and torment one examination discovered it to help in recuperating Achilles tendinitis, typical foot damage; another refered to positive outcomes when utilized on patients with osteoarthritis.

Dr. Lorenc additionally says red light treatment advances snappier recuperating time for wounds and diminishes post-exercise aggravation. More on that here: The Benefits of Red, Green, and Blue Light Therapy

Are there any reactions of red light treatment?

"It's totally noninvasive and alright for everybody," says Vargas. Not at all like numerous different lasers utilized on the skin, (for example, an IPL, or extreme heartbeat light) that reason harm to instigate tissue fix, red light treatment makes zero harm the skin. "Individuals frequently botch light for laser, or feel that red light treatment will cause affectability, yet it doesn't."

In addition, Vargas considers red to be treatment as a significant type of treatment, not just a delight treatment. In 2014, the diary Photomedicine and Laser Surgery took a gander at both collagen creation and emotional patient fulfillment. Regardless of a little example size (around 200 subjects), most subjects experienced essentially improved skin composition and skin feeling, alongside an expansion in ultrasonographically estimated collagen thickness. Not exclusively was facial skin took a gander at, however the whole body, with correspondingly improved skin composition results.

Where would you be able to attempt red light treatment?

In case you're willing to dish out genuine dollars, you can buy a full-body red light treatment bed for your home as much as $3,000. You can likewise visit a spa. For instance, Vargas' namesake spa offers, LED light treatment medications for face and body beginning at $150 for 30 minutes.

Be that as it may, you can likewise securely attempt red light treatment without making a beeline for your derm's office with cool facial contraptions and apparatuses, the best of which accompany a FDA blessing. Dr. Lorenc really built up the adored Neutrogena Acne Light Mask, which utilizes both blue light treatment to eliminate microorganisms and red light treatment to decrease irritation all from the solace of your own home. "Not just has the cover demonstrated to be successful in the treatment of kindled skin break out, but on the other hand it's delicate enough on skin to be utilized every day," he includes. (Related: Can At-Home Blue Light Devices Really Clear Acne?)

Step by Step Guide to red therapy

Imagine having the option to improve each conceivable skin worry, from skin break out to wrinkles—alongside balding, wounds and diseases—with zero personal time, symptoms or security concerns.

In all honesty, you can, with red light treatment!

In Part 1 of this meeting with light master Joe Hollins-Gibson, we discussed what red light treatment involves, and the key skin, hair and wellbeing conditions it can treat.

Joe is the originator of Red Light Man, a retailer spend significant time in incredible, cutting edge light gadgets. In the event that you missed Part 1, look at it here.

Red Light Man sells powerful light treatment gadgets for home and expert use.

There are likewise full-body LED light beds at different spas. Joanna Vargas was one of the primary estheticians to put resources into one, which you can lie in for $300 per 75-minute session. Not modest either!

At that point there are the hand-held light devices from

brands, for example, Baby Quasar, LightStim, Silk'n, Skin Inc. furthermore, NuFace, which are progressively reasonable however tedious to utilize.

These choices are great... in any case, in the event that you ask me, you can improve.

I propose searching for a red light that conveys logically demonstrated wavelengths of light; at a powerful thickness (with the goal that medications take insignificant minutes); that you can use at home as frequently as you like.

That is the reason I'm educating you regarding Red Light Man. (Not supported, I just really have confidence in these gadgets and Joe's ability!)

In Part 2, beneath, you'll discover:

- The distinction between red light and infrared light, and which one to pick
- How red light looks at to different shades of light (counting blue) and IPL
- Why most red light gadgets—even the Déesse!— aren't successful
- What to search for in a red light and the best gadgets to treat different skin and hair concerns

- The most effective method to utilize your gadget at home for best outcomes
- The most effective method to get 10 percent off at Red Light Man!

Red Light versus Infrared Light

Red Light Man Infrared Light Device (left) and Red Light Device (right). Note: These are more established models; both currently come in the square configuration.

You sell both Red and Infrared light gadgets. What's the distinction?

The most evident distinction is that red light (600 to 700 nm) is obvious and brilliant, though infrared or close infrared light (700 to 900 nm) is non-noticeable and must be seen as a black out warmth on the skin.

As far as the restorative properties, red light is assimilated very well by the skin, making it helpful for any treatment there, just as the treatment of the hair.

Infrared light is increasingly penetrative. It can

possibly treat the tissue underneath the skin—joints, bones, muscles, and so forth.— in spite of the fact that it is as yet retained in the skin to a noteworthy degree and gives benefits there.

It is safe to say that one is superior to the next?

It isn't so much that one is superior to the next, just maybe increasingly suitable for specific conditions and body parts.

In principle, you can utilize it is possible that one for basically any skin condition.

Red light appears to be favored for things like burn from the sun, skin inflammation, male pattern baldness, wound mending, yeast contaminations, general enemy of maturing, etc. Studies contrasting the two kinds of light appear to show comparative outcomes, however.

Would it be gainful to utilize both red and infrared lights to get greatest outcomes?

It's certainly valuable to have both accessible.

It's critical to realize that close infrared light enters

far superior to red light, maybe around multiple times better to the more profound tissue.

On the off chance that you're just keen on the skin, at that point you will approve of a red light.

Be that as it may, in the event that you are keen on different advantages to more profound tissue like muscles, joints and bones, at that point you ought to consider getting an infrared light, or both.

Red Light versus Different Colors

The Foreo Espada treats skin inflammation with blue light, which can quicken maturing.

You referenced that red light can help with skin inflammation. In any case, I've just at any point seen blue light gadgets sold for that reason, (for example, the Foreo Espada). Why?

Solid blue light has a disinfecting impact on microbes, including skin inflammation.

It includes some significant pitfalls, however, as blue light damages our very own cells, as well. Studies show it is powerful against skin break out for the time being, yet it additionally expands our pace of maturing and harms our visual perception, among other negative impacts.

So would you propose maintaining a strategic distance from blue light?

Red light is demonstrated to be compelling against skin break out and has no negative symptoms, settling on it a superior decision.

Shouldn't something be said about different shades of light, for example, green and golden? Gadgets like the Déesse include all these various shades.

Green and golden are not too contemplated as red and blue, and don't deal with similar systems, albeit a lot of information exists. They have a wide scope of impacts on various pieces of the body because of how they respond with colors in our cells. Nonetheless, they do not have the vitality boosting and mending impacts of red light treatment.

Melanin in our skin, for instance, has a wide retention range (500 to 1,100 nm), retaining green, yellow, orange, red and close infrared light. So green and golden can be useful in things like hyperpigmentation—however so can red, and red enters better.

These hues are utilized in different treatments like colourpuncture and shading treatment, however they don't have indistinguishable direct advantages to the skin from red and infrared light.

The other wavelength run that gives direct fundamental advantages is bright B (UVB), which helps nutrient D creation and decreases resistant reactions in the skin for things like psoriasis. Be that as it may, UV light can prompt skin harm.

What's your supposition on light medicines, for example, IPL (serious beat light)? Could individuals get practically identical outcomes at home with red light treatment?

I don't think IPL is an equivalent kind of treatment to red light treatment—the two of them utilize light however are altogether different in instrument. Be that as it may, IPL is a powerful treatment for things like skin pigmentation and hair evacuation. Red light won't expel undesirable hair.

For most different issues, IPL is a significant savage

power technique to accomplish what red or infrared light treatment will accomplish in an increasingly characteristic manner.

On the off chance that you are on an IPL treatment course, it's great to utilize red or close infrared light previously as well as after the medications to help diminish the symptoms and speed recuperating.

The most effective method to Choose a Red Light Therapy Device

The four best "tops" of light are 620 nm, 670 nm, 760 nm and 830 nm (+/ - 15 nm). (Source: Red Light Man)

Is there an ideal wavelength scope of red light that individuals should search for in a gadget?

The general scope of light utilized in red light treatment is somewhere in the range of 600 and 900 nm, here and there higher. You can get profits by any wavelength between those qualities.

Passing by the examinations on wavelength viability (T. Karu et al.), our cells ingest and utilize 4 "tops" of light superior to the others: 620 nm, 670 nm, 760 nm and 830 nm, +/ - 15 nm. Those are the wavelengths you should attempt to get.

Qualities in the middle of those pinnacle esteems, for example, 645 nm or 720 nm, might be under 50 percent as compelling, albeit still helpful.

Close however not impeccable wavelengths, for example, 660 nm, 810 nm and others are demonstrated helpful.

How significant is the power of the light?

The range that appears to be successful in thinks about is between 20 to 200 mW/cm², with 100 to 200 mW/cm² being more for infrared light treatment on more profound tissue, and 20 to 100 mW/cm² for red light on the skin.

Are most light gadgets available conveying these qualities?

Most other light treatment items available simply utilize the least expensive and most promptly accessible wavelengths, for example, 660 nm or 850 nm. Or then again surprisingly more terrible, they utilize less viable wavelengths like 650 nm or 880 nm.

A great deal of gadgets I have seen are likewise amazingly frail, with most extreme power densities around the 10 mW/cm² imprint or more regrettable—which means they may never be viable, or you need to utilize them for exceptionally long session times, in any event, when squeezed legitimately onto the skin.

What makes your Red Light Man gadgets better?

We're utilizing the precise wavelengths saw as the best at animating our cells: 620 nm, 670 nm, 760 nm and 830nm.

Our gadgets all yield up to in any event 200 mW/cm², so you can simply modify the separation to change your treatment times—further away for lower light force and longer sessions (covering a bigger surface zone).

Red Light Man Devices

Which of your gadgets would you suggest for somebody who is simply beginning with light treatment?

I think the mix lights we offer, including both red and close infrared LEDs, are the best decision to begin.

You can utilize them on essentially any condition, be it somewhere down in the body or quite shallow.

The Red-Infrared Combo Mini is our most well known item.

Red Light Man Red-Infrared Combo Mini

We additionally sell the Combo Light, which is progressively exceptional.

Red Light Man Red-Infrared Combo Light

Would the Combo Light be as ground-breaking as utilizing Red and Infrared lights independently?

Our principle Combo Light is practically a similar power as our primary Red or Infrared units, yes. You can see the thickness readings here:

Red Light Man gadget control thickness examination.

So you can see that the Combo is more fragile

regarding completely vitality yield, yet the more tightly bar edge empowers the light power to convey a further separation. The 200 mW/cm² is commonly the top furthest reaches of intensity thickness you'll find in thinks about, so the entirety of the models are effectively ground-breaking enough to coordinate any investigation convention.

The Combo is, obviously, a blend of half red and half infrared, however since it is all following up on the equivalent mitochondrial instrument, everything considers the equivalent (other than the distinctions in entrance).

I think the higher densities are valuable for that more profound entrance you have to see impacts in joints, muscles, and so on.

In the event that you can stand to put resources into discrete Red and Infrared gadgets, would that be surprisingly better?

I think the Combo is the best decision on the off chance that somebody can just bear the cost of one light, yet the different gadgets are progressively ideal generally speaking.

Red Light Man Red Light Device

For instance, on the off chance that you are utilizing the Combo light for joints, the red light it yields is nearly squandered, simply being consumed by the skin, while the infrared will arrive at the joint tissue. Despite the fact that the Combo will even now work, it would be better and increasingly effective to utilize an unadulterated Infrared for that.

Red Light Man Infrared Light Device

I don't think the Combo is basic on the off chance that you can manage the cost of the two separate Red and Infrared gadgets.

What are the best alternatives on the off chance that you explicitly need to treat the skin surface?

For skin maturing and pigmentation, search for wavelengths close to either 610 to 630 nm or 670 nm.

The Red Mini 670 is our most prominent light for skin medicines.

Red Light Man Red Mini 670

For pigmentation, I would utilize something like the Red Light Device Mini, which produces 610 nm, 630 nm and 670 nm.

Red Light Man Red Light Device Mini

For skin inflammation, I would utilize a ground-breaking item like the Red Light Device.

Shouldn't something be said about somebody who needs to get most extreme outcomes—what would it be a good idea for them to put resources into?

Full body treatment is certainly the best approach on the off chance that you need the greatest outcomes. Our full body light is so amazing, it tends to be utilized from up to two meters away.

Red Light Man Combo Bodylight 2.0

Red Light Therapy for Hair Loss

The Red Light Man Infrared Light Device is perfect for treating balding, among different issues. (Note: This is a more seasoned model; it presently comes in the square organization.)

You referenced that red light treatment can help

with male pattern baldness. What's your opinion of the laser tops or head protectors available for this reason?

A laser top or protective cap appears from the outset like a decent.

There are numerous advantages an individual can get with red light treatment nonetheless, it can get expensive to go to a salon or spa and experience red light treatment in a few sessions. Why not purchase your very own at-home red light treatment gadget and offer the light with the remainder of your family? We recorded down the advantages of utilizing red light treatment and why it is a wise venture

Red Light Therapy Benefits

Red Light Therapy is 100% regular, concoction free and medication free medium to battle indications of maturing. Not at all like concoction arrangements or toners that you apply on your skin, the normal red light utilized in the LED light enters the skin to initiate cell movement. You don't need to give your skin a chance to leak each one of those synthetic compounds that over the long haul, can be lethal for you.

red light treatment machine

It is an easy, non-ablative and non-obtrusive technique. All you need is to relax under the light and let it help produce fibroblasts and collagen to address indications of skin maturing. No compelling reason to go under the blade or torment yourself with needles. It doesn't harm the skin and it requires zero personal time. All you need is 5 minutes and you can approach your day, apply cosmetics, get down to business or go out with your companions without stressing that your skin will look awful.

This light treatment is ok for all skin types and has no known unfriendly reactions. This well-inquired about at-home red light treatment gadget is FDA-endorsed to treat full facial wrinkles. It is alright for all ages. Individuals with a restricted scope of movement or physical handicap and the older may require help with working the gadget.

Treatment for Your Skin

Red light treatment enters various degrees of the

skin to energize cell movement and increment blood supply to the skin's surface. Expanded blood stream to the region implies more supplements and oxygen to sustain the skin cells. This additionally prompts the generation of fibroblasts and collagen that guides in the redress and counteractive action of certain skin issues.

The utilization of red light treatment brings about a more advantageous and gleaming skin and accomplishes a smoother skin tone. It amends sun harm procured through long periods of disregard.

Expanded blood stream likewise lessens barely recognizable differences and wrinkles. It works extraordinary in decreasing Crow's feet and it relax chuckle lines and temple wrinkles as well!

Trophy Skin

It likewise hurries the skin's capacity to mend flaws like skin inflammation or little cuts or scratches. Beside that, it likewise underpins the fix and making of vessels to diminish flushing or redness. Red light treatment additionally fixes and helps stretch checks and scars.

Utilizations of Red Light Therapy

Since Red light treatment can assist speed with increasing the skin's capacity to mend, it very well may be utilized to address various issues including the accompanying:

Skin break out and Inflamed Acne Marks. Albeit Red Light isn't utilized to slaughter skin break out causing microscopic organisms, it will help lessen the irritation achieved by skin inflammation. Red and Infrared lights enter the skin at various levels and catalyst the cells to fix the skin from inside. It fixes the skin tissues that skin break out has decimated. This prompts quicker mending of the skin break out and counteracts further tissue harm that may prompt setting skin break out scars. Then again, Blue Light Therapy is clinically demonstrated to starve off P. acnes microscopic organisms that is the most well-known reason for skin break out.

Chomps. Due to the red light's capacity to accelerate recuperating, nibble wounds or punctures to the skin will be mended quicker due to expanded blood stream to the region.

Wounds. Wounds are brought about by spilling blood to the skin tissues either by an immediate injury or broken vessels. Since the blood can't leave the body with no break to the skin, it emits a somewhat blue shade that is the thing that we regularly call a wound. Red light treatment will have the option to convey supplement rich blood supply to the region quicker that will fix and help in the development of new vessels.

Minor Burns. Red Light Therapy doesn't radiate warmth so it won't add to the harm that consumes cause. What it will do is increment the blood supply to the territory with the goal that our body's characteristic guards and fix component will have the option to do its work quicker.

Cuts, Scrapes and Wound Care. Like referenced, expanded blood stream to the region assists speed with increasing the body's capacity to fix itself normally.

Dry Skin and Psoriasis. The Red Light infiltrates the thickened skin and catalyst the skin cells. In view of the expanded blood stream to the outside of the skin being dealt with, more supplements are conveyed to that territory. That implies it extinguishes the thirst of the skin to be sustained. Oxygen-rich blood streams to the treated regions, additionally expanding the hydration achieved by great blood supply.

Scars and Stretch imprints. Stretch imprints are realized by droopy skin either from weight reduction or maturing. Collagen exhaustion from the body brings about having free, stretchy and droopy skin. Red light treatment invigorates collagen generation in this manner averting further advancement of stretch imprints. It additionally helps and reduce scars and even by and large skin tone.

Sun Damage. Red light is a whiz in remedying sun harm. Sans uv LED bulbs are utilized to securely and successfully convey red light treatment. The red light wavelength spikes cell movement to assist switch with sunning harm. It can help age spots.

Wrinkles. Due to loss of collagen, wrinkles begin to crawl up all over (or neck). Red light treatment helps support collagen and fibroblasts generation to help right these unattractive indications of maturing. It deals with undereye wrinkles, temple wrinkles, chuckle lines, and crow's feet. RejuvaliteMD from Trophy Skin is FDA-endorsed to treat full facial wrinkles.

Treatment for Pain and Injury

Red light treatment accelerates the recuperating of wounds and wounds to the body and decreases aggravation as well. It can improve the scope of movement of joints which is a typical issue for the individuals who are encountering joint inflammation, back torment, carpal passage disorder, and different types of joint agonies. It decreases torment for the individuals who endure fibromyalgia as well.

Animates Hair Growth

Beside taking a shot at the skin, it works for the hair as well! You needn't bother with laser lights to invigorate your hair follicle to develop. The correct sort of red light wavelength is sufficient to kick off hair development!

There are numerous variables to consider in the accomplishment of regrowing hair. The key is to have noticeable red light consumed by the hair follicle. Wavelengths between 630-670 nanometers are best in being retained and cause a characteristic organic response to animate hair development.

Presently, if the hair follicle has really passed on, it can't ingest the unmistakable red light. Really awful there are no realized medications to restore dead hair follicles yet.

Accomplishment in regrowing hair additionally depends on how early the treatment is begun. The previous that it is done, the better the outcomes. The sort of male pattern baldness matters as well.

Red light male pattern baldness treatments are suggested for people who have impermanent male pattern baldness because of issues, for example, prescription reactions, stress, medical procedure, or other male pattern baldness conditions, for example, male example hair loss or menopause.

Presently, don't stress that it will cause hair development in undesirable regions. In the event that no hair follicles are available in the regions you will treat, at that point no hair will develop there. It won't thicken your facial hair.

It takes around 2 to 3 months to see huge outcomes in red light treatment for hair regrow. Be quiet and remember to do your medications every day for best outcomes.

Treatment for Rosacea

This medication free and compound free treatment have no announced reactions which settle on it a reasonable decision of treatment for rosacea. It is non-obtrusive and is alright for day by day use.

Noticeable red light can help the skin's capacity to recuperate itself by 200%. The skin assimilates the red light which can control up the skin cells to recuperate itself. It can improve blood stream to convey oxygen to regions that need fix and mend harm.

Since red light can enter the skin, it can recuperate rosacea-related skin break out without the utilization of synthetic substances that make the skin additional touchy. It has no personal time and is a protected and easy approach to treat rosacea.

The various wavelengths of red light utilized in RejuvaliteMD are powerful in diminishing irritation and lessen redness, growing and skin delicacy. It can oversee redness or flushing and support the recuperating of the skin from inside.

Red Light Therapy for Losing Weight

In spite of the fact that it sounds difficult to get in shape by simply sparkling red lights on greasy territories of the body, it is sponsored by science. Red Light makes it simpler for individuals to get thinner since it makes fat cells dump their substance, making fats simpler to be expelled by the body.

At the point when red light is utilized on fat tissues, it makes the fats separate. Fats are then changed over to carbon dioxide which we expel from our body through peeing, crapping and breathing out.

You don't require incredible lasers to impact and evacuate fat cells. You additionally don't have to experience liposuction and different medical procedures to expel abundance fats. Indeed, even the straightforward LED's can help in diminishing weight. You simply need the right wavelengths between 630 to 680 nm to take the necessary steps.

Nonetheless, on the off chance that you don't make

the vital way of life changes that will bolster your weight reduction, you won't value your outcomes. In the event that you continue gorging on salty tidbits and lousy nourishment, you will hold progressively fluid and it will make you feel enlarged. Undesirable eating additionally adds more to body fats and weight gain.

In fact, red light treatment can be utilized in numerous medical issues identified with the skin and different pieces of the body. It is a wise venture since it can address stylish issues, yet it has likewise been demonstrated to hurry wound fix, reduce torment, develop hair back, oversee rosacea, shed pounds and delay the maturing procedure.

Presently the main inquiry remains, does red light treatment work? Assuming this is the case, how does this innovation work?

Does Red Light Therapy Work

NASA pondered something very similar! So they dispatched QDI to direct research on red light treatment in 1993. After it was demonstrated that the innovation could enact plant development in space, they at that point started to examine the restorative use of LEDs with a unique spotlight on how LED vitality moves to human cells. The exploration exhibited the successful medical advantages of a particular wavelength of red light: 660 nanometers (nm). What started as an approach to confine the bone and muscle loss of space travelers at that point prompted many companion surveyed clinical examinations recording a wide assortment of advantages. Indeed, even the FDA has endorsed light treatment for the treatment of joint torment and joint inflammation, decrease of wrinkles and numerous different conditions.

Red Light Therapy

Advantages of Red Light Therapy

How Does Red Light Therapy Work

Not at all like numerous different kinds of treatment red light treatment is totally protected and non-obtrusive. It utilizes no synthetic concoctions and has no destructive symptoms. It very well may be utilized on all skin types. RLT utilizes the normal recuperating and restoring advantages of a particular scope of light and conveys this vitality at a higher rate than the sun (without hurtful UV beams).

Need something more specialized? Here ya go… Red light treatment is not quite the same as laser or serious beat light (IPL) treatments since it doesn't make harm the skin surface. Laser and beat light treatments work by making controlled harm the external layer of the skin, which at that point instigates tissue fix. RLT sidesteps this cruel advance by legitimately invigorating recovery of the skin. The light transmitted by RLT enters approximately 5 millimeters underneath the skin's surface. By expanding the capacity of the mitochondria a cell can make more ATP (an unpredictable, natural substance that gives vitality to forms in living cells). With more vitality, cells can work all the more effectively, revive themselves and fix harm.

With respect to how LED Facial Masks explicitly work, I discovered it is normally really, which you all realize I love! Here I will explicitly reference the LED Fast Facial Mask I use. We realize that as we age the skin's collagen and elastin generation eases back. This LED Facial Mask is without uv and contains red and infrared LEDs that work together to improve the presence of temple wrinkles, grin lines, nasal folds and facial structure, just as lines around the mouth and lips (ummm, yes please)!

Advantages Of Red Light Therapy

- Decreases Deep Wrinkles
- Improves Skin Elasticity
- Improves Skin Firmness
- Improves Elasticity of Collagen Fibers
- Decreases Inflammation
- Improves Blood Flow
- Decreases Joint Stiffness
- Eases Muscle Spasms

Benefits of red light therapy

WHAT ARE THE BENEFITS OF RED LIGHT THERAPY?

Red light treatment works from the back to front to improve mitochondrial work in cells. This, thus, prompts a few skin benefits. Red light diminishes skin aggravation, smooths skin tone, fixes sun harm, blurs scars and stretch checks, and even forms collagen in the skin, which decreases wrinkles. It likewise mends wounds and can avoid repeating mouth blisters or herpes simplex. Red light takes a shot at the lymphatic framework to improve your body's detoxification capacities by expanding blood stream. It might even invigorate hair development in your hair follicles.

Studies uncover that red light recuperates age-related macular degeneration of the eyes.[1][2] It's likewise used to treat knee osteoarthritis, hypothyroidism, psychological brokenness following mind damage, and fibromyalgia.

In a scene of Bulletproof Radio (iTunes), Scott Nelson, author of Joov shared the consequences of an investigation including Joov gadgets, indicating the wide range of hormone benefits.

"With the utilization of day by day, full-body red and close infrared light treatment with our gadgets, in addition to the fact that [women] saw extremely solid progesterone increments, however they additionally observed adjusted progesterone to estrogen proportions, which is extremely significant, on the grounds that estrogen strength is extremely regular as females age," says Nelson.

Look at the remainder of the webcast scene to discover how Joov lights expanded testosterone, as well.

WHAT ARE THE BEST SOURCES OF RED LIGHT THERAPY?

You can experience red light treatment with a certified proficient like a prepared rheumatologist or dermatologist. Approach your PCP for a referral.

Some medicinal spas offer red light treatment for about $50-100 for every session. Infrared saunas are extraordinary from normal saunas in that they heat the body from the back to front. Both red light treatment and infrared saunas upgrade mitochondrial work, however in various ways. In contrast to red light treatment, infrared sauna light is obvious – however it enters a lot further into the body. You'll need to examination to see which works best for you. Become familiar with the advantages of infrared sauna use here.

Receive the rewards of red light at home with a light treatment gadget like Joovv. Or then again, introduce red lights around your home – there are red lights on Amazon that sell for as meager as $6. Use them in the early morning and later around evening time, just as restoratively to increment mitochondrial capacity and collagen generation. Hold the light over damage for a couple of moments daily. You can likewise discover LED shaded lights with a brilliance and shading remote controller. (This gives you a chance to change from blue to red, contingent upon what time of day it is.)

The freshest expansion to the red light family is really getting it from your PC or telephone screen. Shading Tint is another element on the Apple iOS 10 that turns your whole screen red, which Apple notes has its own advantages. While they are not really all wellbeing related like a red light treatment box, it is conceivable that you'll squint less taking a gander at your screen in the night because of the red light.

The Science Behind Red Light Therapy

There are in excess of 3,000 friend checked on logical examinations indicating extraordinary wellbeing and hostile to maturing advantages of red light and NIR light treatment, with no known negative reactions (source).

Our bodies are extremely receptive to the nearness and nonattendance of light. It is a direct result of light that we realize when to wake up and rest. It's the fundamental fixing to the generation of essential supplements and synthetic substances inside us. In any case, not all lights on the electromagnetic field are as useful for your wellbeing as red light has all the earmarks of being. The electromagnetic range is comprised of vitality.

Various wavelengths of light encourage or brief diverse real responses — with certain responses superior to other people. At the extraordinary parts of the bargains range dwell unsafe wavelengths, for example, X-beams, gamma beams, and electromagnetic frequencies (EMFs). In the center, however, are wavelengths that contain mending properties.

Each tone of light is one of a kind in the impacts it can deliver. So red light doesn't do indistinguishable things from white, blue, or green lights and the other way around. Being presented to red light initiates a compound response inside our cells that gives the mitochondria control. Cells contain chromophores that produce vitality when they ingest red and infrared light that the mitochondria would then be able to use to work.

At the point when energized, the mitochondria make vitality atoms known as ATP (adenosine triphosphate). At the point when cells have a wealth of ATP available to them, cells can work all the more proficiently, which implies capacities like harm fix and safe capacity in addition to other things are performed far better.

The Benefits of Red Light Therapy

Red light animates both the working of fibroblasts and our dissemination to help in quicker twisted fix times. That is the reason this treatment has been utilized to treat wounds, for example, consumes, contaminated wounds, and removal wounds to guarantee a higher achievement rate for mending. Something else fibroblasts are liable for is the creation of collagen.

Regular daylight is a mix of the whole obvious light range (400-700 nm) just as bright (UV; 300-400 nm) and infrared (700-1000 nm) light. The vast majority are very much aware of the potential perils of an excessive amount of daylight because of harming UV beams. Be that as it may, the body has explicit positive reactions to light in the 600-900 nm wavelength go, likewise called the "remedial window".

Light on the electromagnetic range

This light vitality can go through human tissue a lot simpler than different wavelengths. In particular, light in the mid-600 nm and mid-800 nm run has been appeared to give ideal natural reactions.

This vitality is consumed by the body and animates adenosine triphosphate (ATP), the method of compound vitality transportation at the cell level. As such, cells that get this restoring, hostile to maturing jolt of energy can play out their common capacities at an increased level (source).

A portion of the reported advantages of light treatment include:

- Improved skin tone and appearance
- Improved invulnerable framework work
- Invigorated generation of collagen and elastin –

we consolidate red light treatment with drinking collagen peptides

- Improved muscle recuperation and athletic execution
- Enhanced cerebrum and intellectual capacity; builds neuroprotection
- Decreased joint agony, aggravation, and joint pain
- Improved appearance of wrinkles, scarcely discernible differences, and stretch imprints
- Decreased skin break out, rosacea, and dermatitis
- Expanded flow
- Quicker mending of wounds and wounds

At the point when your fibroblasts are presented to red light, they make more collagen also. Collagen makes up the greater part of the protein found in our skin, so by having a greater amount of it present, wrinkles, stretch lines, and other skin imperfections start to blur and turn out to be less recognizable.

Red light treatment treats other skin conditions too, for example, psoriasis. One examination found that individuals with psoriasis who were treated with NIR and red light treatment saw critical outcomes due to approach infrared's calming nature and red light's capacity to recuperate wounds rapidly. This aggravation help additionally mitigates joint agony from conditions, for example, joint pain.

Where would you be able to get red light treatment?

Red light treatment is rapidly getting generally accessible through specialist's workplaces, restorative spas, wellness studios and at-home treatment units. One of the regions where red light treatment has increased noteworthy footing in the biohacking scene. Genuine beginner competitors and extreme C-suite executives are consistently looking for that additional edge to put their exhibition over the top, and cutting edge half and half wellness and bio-hacking focuses, for example, Upgrade Labs are rapidly jumping up to fulfill the need. Situated in Los Angeles, Upgrade Labs is the brainchild of Bulletproof espresso maker Dave Asprey and offers a large group of treatments and medications, including red light treatment

"From a wellness point of view, red light animates more vitality (at a phone level) so you can feel more grounded, longer during your exercises," says Amanda

McVey, VP Experience and Programming. "Red light likewise builds blood flow, lessen expanding and irritation. This implies you'll recoup all the more rapidly after a serious exercise."

Wellness studios committed to amplifying your time spent perspiring in class are touting offices decked out with red light boards to upgrade execution and recuperation, for example, Red Effect Infrared Fitness.

Who utilizes red light treatment?

The energy for red light treatment arrived at the pined for domain of the Hollywood A-List blessing pack this spring. Different at-home red light treatment units were included not long ago in the select and spendy swag packs for chosen people and participants during the current year's Hollywood honor show season.

Sweat Sauna was the main infrared sauna studio in the U.S., and CEO Lee Braun shares, "Sweat Sauna Studio has had a couple of VIPs come into our studios for infrared and shading light treatment sessions, including Andre 3000 (of Outkast), Ludacris, and Ireland Baldwin. Kim Kardashian has been exceptionally imminent about her battles with psoriasis and how light treatment has been one of the main successful methods for recuperating it."

Kanye West additionally disclosed to David Letterman that he explicitly utilizes red light treatment in his exhibitions as an advantage to the group of spectators: "They maneuver you into a Zen space, and to reconstruct ... to be increasingly quiet, at the time to be progressively steady.'"

Furthermore, shouldn't something be said about those extravagant at-home packs that the Hollywood set was given this spring—do they really work?

"At-home LED gadgets can give comparative advantages, anyway they ordinarily don't have the full quality of expert machines. This implies you would require progressively customary home medicines to accomplish a comparable impact," Desko says. "To guarantee the best outcomes from your at-home treatment, the light ought to be aimed at the skin persistently for 15-20 minutes, so a LED light veil is a superior choice than a handheld gadget that you need to move consistently over the skin. Another key factor to search for is the quantity of LED lights in the machine. For the most part the higher the quantity of bulbs, the more grounded the impact. The quantity of LED bulbs additionally by and large matches with gadget cost, so be set up to compensation extra for a higher quality machine."

It's significant that Neutrogena as of late pulled its red light treatment cover off the market because of worries that wearing the veil mistakenly might cause eye damage. You can in any case purchase the brand's wand type of the treatment, the Red and Blue Light Acne Spot Treatment.

Similarly as with any health practice, make certain to check with your primary care physician before beginning anything new to ensure it's a solid match for you. Los Angeles-based, board-confirmed dermatologist Tsippora Shainhouse, MD, of SkinSafe Dermatology and Skin Care offers a few hints for when to utilize red light treatment underneath:

- It very well may be utilized after progressively forceful skin medications (strips, facials, extractions, lasers, dermabrasion, and so forth.) to speed skin fix.
- It is utilized in patients accepting chemotherapy who have agonizing skin sloughing in the oral

mucosa (mouth) to help speed mending.

- It might help twisted recuperating in diabetic skin ulcers, when utilized related to other treatment modalities.
- It can help invigorate new hair development in patients with androgenic alopecia. Tops and looks over are accessible for home utilize 3-7 days per week to animate and "empower" the undifferentiated organisms in the hair follicle to energize new hair development.
- It very well may be utilized as a component of a home skincare routine 1-2 times each week to conceivably help calm and treat aggravated or treated skin.

Instruments

A large portion of red light's belongings are through the cells' mitochondria retaining light. In cell thinks about, the cytochrome c oxidase in the mitochondria ingests red light, which makes it discharge nitric oxide, increment ATP, and abatement oxidative pressure

As per a few scientists, this would then be able to cause a chain response in the cells and influence reactions, for example, cell arrangement, development, demise, and aggravation. Be that as it may, its impacts rely upon the kind of cell and its status

This expanded ATP (vitality) generation is a potential reason for light treatment's constructive outcomes on muscle recuperation and physical execution.

Potential Health Benefits

While there are FDA-endorsed red light gadgets, these are comprehensively delegated class 2 gadgets; that is, while there is proof to help their utilization in some wellbeing conditions (which we'll talk about in this area), they are as of now not adequately managed to ensure the viability or security of a specific gadget.

On the off chance that you are keen on utilizing red light treatment, we prescribe conversing with your primary care physician to pick the correct gadget and decide if this technique is directly for you.

Likely Effective For

1) Skin Quality

In an investigation of 31 subjects, a blend of red and infrared LED light treatment improved skin conditions.

They had less sun-initiated maturing and wrinkles.

In a DB-RCT of 52 female patients, 12 weeks of every day treatment with red light treatment fundamentally improved eye wrinkles.

A comparable report indicated that LED treatment is compelling against sunspots in moderately aged members.

In a solitary blinded RCT, red light was better than infrared light in treating skin break out .

The expansion of red light to blue light likewise improved skin break out side effects fundamentally contrasted with blue light alone and benzoyl peroxide in a RCT of 107 skin break out patients .

Red light treatment likewise altogether improved skin appearance, harshness, and collagen thickness in a RCT of 136 members.

Notwithstanding, in human cells, a few qualities related with skin scarring expanded with red light like receptive oxygen species and collagen development restraint.

Conceivably Effective For

2) Oral Mucositis

A typical symptom of chemotherapy is oral mucositis, which is when aggravation separates the coating of the mouth. In an efficient audit of 11 RCTs, both red and infrared light treatment fundamentally decreased the rate and seriousness of oral mucositis .

3) Bipolar Disorder

A survey of numerous sorts of light treatment discovered red light treatment improved burdensome manifestations and forestalled backslide after lack of sleep in patients with bipolar issue .

4) Physical Performance

In an investigation of 39 coronary illness patients, red light treatment improved execution and diminished chest torment during exercise tests.

In a DB-RCT, 40 solid untrained men experienced an escalated exercise session. The members that experienced red light treatment had fundamentally improved execution, diminished irritation, and decreased markers of muscle harm contrasted with ones that didn't have light treatment.

In female competitors, 2 weeks of red light treatment improved rest quality and continuance.

Red light treatment additionally altogether improved recuperation after high-power practice in a DB-RCT of 40 volunteers .

Strikingly, these outcomes have made analysts question whether it ought to be allowed in athletic rivalries because of its viability in upgrading athletic execution and improving recuperation.

Inadequate Evidence For

The accompanying implied benefits are just bolstered by restricted, low-quality clinical investigations. There is deficient proof to help the utilization of red light treatment for any of the underneath recorded employments. Make sure to talk with a specialist before utilizing red light treatment, and it ought to never be utilized to supplant something your primary care physician has suggested or endorsed.

5) Wound Healing

In a triple-dazzle RCT of 12 dental patients, red light treatment improved the mending rate after oral medical procedure. In any case, it didn't decrease torment.

In a RCT of 16 diabetic patients, red light treatment essentially diminished diabetic foot ulcer size and decreased torment .

Another RCT of 30 diabetic patients indicated comparative outcomes; red light treatment joined with regular treatment diminished ulcer size more than customary treatment alone.

In diabetic rodent models of skin wound and consume damage, red light altogether improved recuperating and was better than infrared treatment for consume wounds.

Red light additionally upgraded the mending pace of cut injuries in diabetic rodents and decreased the danger of disease.

In bunnies with skin wounds, red light treatment diminished recuperating time fundamentally more than blue light or no light treatment. It advanced tissue and cell development.

6) Inflammation

One of the principle employments of red light treatment is to treat irritation.

Red light treatment confines the fiery reaction and diminishes oxidative harm by decreasing incendiary cytokines (TNF-an, IL-1A, and IL-6).

An audit on muscle fix (in creature models) inferred that red light treatment has the ability to decrease aggravation, decidedly sway development factors, and increment vein arrangement.

7) Pain

In an examination (DB-RCT) of 80 chemotherapy patients, red light altogether decreased self-detailed torment .

Red light treatment may treat tennis elbow for a brief timeframe, yet these discoveries were just appeared by one examination (RCT).

As to interminable low back torment, discoveries are blended.

In mice, red LED treatment diminished torment and improved movement after spinal rope damage .

8) Cognitive Function

Red light treatment has been considered in a wide

assortment of conditions including stroke, Alzheimer's, and Parkinson's malady, melancholy, and intellectual improvement in sound subjects.

In a DB-RCT of 11 dementia patients, red and close infrared light treatment improved memory, consideration, and official capacity.

In one contextual investigation, red light treatment likewise diminished despondency, nervousness, cerebral pain, and a sleeping disorder. Then, their psychological capacity and personal satisfaction improved.

Red light treatment may likewise improve mind work after awful cerebrum damage. In two contextual analyses, red light treatment improved memory, consideration, and even diminished PTSD in one patient

In rodents, red light treatment adjusted fiery marker levels (IL-1β, TNF-α, and IL-6) and anticipated cell demise. This improved cerebrum work for about a month after head damage.

9) Antimicrobial Activity

In HPV patients, 3 months of red light treatment

additionally killed the human papillomavirus from their body. Be that as it may, it is conceivable to be re-tainted after light treatment is done .

In dental patients, red light treatment can help decrease diseases and irritation during oral medical procedure.

Red light eliminated microscopic organisms (Propionibacterium acnes, Actinomyces odontolyticus, and Porphyromonas gingivalis) in plaque tests from dental patients .

10) Hair Growth

In a DB-RCT, red light treatment each other day for 17 weeks actuated hair regrowth in ladies with androgenic alopecia (thinning up top because of hormonal unevenness).

In a DB-RCT of 41 men, red light treatment each other day for about four months essentially expanded hair follicles comparative with fake treatment.

Surveys on alopecia and male pattern baldness finished up red light treatment was sheltered and compelling for the two people.

Symptoms, Caveats, Gene Interactions

There are no announced symptoms of red light treatment. The most widely recognized objection is tiredness and redness of the skin.

All things considered, we prescribe conversing with your primary care physician before endeavoring to utilize red light treatment for any restorative reason, and never use it instead of something your PCP has suggested or recommended.

Admonitions

In spite of the fact that the impacts of red light treatment have been predictable over a wide scope of wound kinds and creature models, enormous clinical preliminaries in people are deficient around there.

Furthermore, the vast majority of the examinations accessible are utilizing laser treatment, not drove boards. Despite the fact that both utilize red light wavelengths, the impacts of lasers and boards might be extraordinary.

Quality Interactions

Red light treatment can increment and lessening the articulation (creation) of numerous qualities. In human cells, by expanding certain quality action, red light helps increment cell arrangement, cancer prevention agent action, and vitality creation.

6 BENEFITS OF RED LIGHT THERAPY

Improved rest

I saw that I began resting better in the wake of utilizing myJoovv™ Light normally. I wasn't exactly certain how this system was functioning, however I went over this passage from the article, The Importance of Natural Sunlight and its Connection to Light Therapy:

Our retinas are associated straightforwardly to the suprachiasmatic cores (SCN) of the body. Along these lines, light got through your eyes assumes a basic job in hormonal capacities—including melatonin creation, which manages our rest. Literally, your body knows to stop this hormone through introduction to morning daylight. This kind of introduction promptly in the day additionally helps produce melatonin later at night, when light is missing.

Getting normal daylight at the correct occasions of the day helps set your circadian mood. You can encounter these advantages by presenting yourself to morning sun (without shades) every day.

For some reasons, this isn't constantly conceivable. You may have constrained daylight where you live or you are simply extremely occupied to go for a stroll each morning. I'm in that pontoon as a single parent, working all day. It would be unimaginable for me to add another progression to our morning schedule in the middle of pressing lunch, appreciating breakfast and preparing everybody for the afternoon.

In the event that you can't get customary daylight toward the beginning of the day, you can encounter the restorative impacts of red and close infrared wavelengths of light by utilizing a quality, full-body, photobiomodulation gadget that gives comparative mending benefits.

Improved state of mind

This advantage is one of the all the more entrancing to me, as it truly shows the association between our bodies and our brains. I notice that my mind-set improves when I routinely utilize my Joovv™ Light. I conversed with a companion that normally utilizes hers as well and she announced comparable outcomes. Studies have indicated that light presentation through our eyes is attached to expanded dopamine generation. Dopamine is a concoction that is controlled by light and discharged in the mind. It works as a synapse and is firmly attached to the feelings of remuneration and joy.

Improved skin

Red and close infrared light have been appeared to invigorate the generation of collagen, which legitimately identifies with the versatility, immovability, and completion of your skin.

Collagen is a long-chain amino corrosive and the most bounteous protein in the body. It's liable for giving skin flexibility, hair its quality, and connective tissue its capacity to hold everything set up. While collagen is advantageous to the whole body, it's most recognizably helpful to the skin. This is on the grounds that as an individual ages, the epidermis (external layer of skin) gets more slender and loses versatility through a procedure called elastosis.

As red light treatment reestablishes solid cell work, it builds the generation of collagen, which thus can smooth wrinkles and improve tone.

At the point when red and close infrared light is consumed by the skin, it animates new skin cells to develop in a more advantageous manner, gives security against harm, and recuperates an assortment of skin issues.

Moreover, red light treatment is thought to improve skin break out on the grounds that it impacts sebum creation, which adds to skin break out.

I've battled with my skin as long as I can remember, even as a grown-up. I encountered a colossal improvement when I tidied up my eating routine and embraced a genuine nourishment way of life. Notwithstanding, my skin scars actually effectively. It appears as though every pimple I've at any point had has left a type of unmistakable imprint. Presently at 37, my skin is at long last looking truly great. This is a photograph taken as of late with no cosmetics on. The elements that have improved my skin all the more as of late are utilizing myJoovv™ Light day by day, one session of microneedling (I am anticipating doing 2 more) and utilizing Beautycounter's Overnight Resurfacing Peel consistently.

Fat Loss

Red light treatment has demonstrated positive outcomes for fat misfortune and body forming over a few diverse clinical investigations. To put it plainly, most analysts concur that light treatment influences adipocytes, which are cells that store fat, making the lipids scatter.

Here is a portion of an examination from the article, The Remarkable Benefits of Red Light Therapy for Weight Loss and Fat Reduction:

An examination in the Journal of Obesity Surgery explored red light treatment for body forming. This 2011 twofold visually impaired, randomized examination performed light treatment at 635-680 nanometers (nm) on members for about a month and recorded consequences for the waistline. Toward the finish of the examination, members had accomplished a measurably noteworthy decrease in waistline circumference.

Expanded Testosterone in Men

A few research articles have bolstered the possibility that uncovering the middle or the testicles to light has been appeared to build testosterone in men. It's essential to utilize a gadget that transmits the right wavelengths with basically no-heat, for example, The Joovv™ Light.

Testosterone is a hormone found in all people, yet ladies produce it in a lot littler sums. Testosterone generation begins to increment essentially during pubescence and starts to plunge after age 30 or somewhere in the vicinity. This is typical, yet it can cause diminished sexual capacity, diminished vitality, a decrease in muscle, and an expansion in fat.

Red light treatment is one characteristic approach to build testosterone. What's more, a decent diet, appropriate rest and lessening pressure may help as well.

Hair Growth

A methodical writing audit assessed eleven examinations, which researched an aggregate of 680 patients, comprising of 444 guys and 236 females. Nine out of 11 examinations evaluating hair check/hair thickness found measurably noteworthy upgrades in the two guys and females following red light treatment.

Other outstanding advantages of Red Light Therapy incorporate muscle tissue fix, blurring of scars and stretch imprints, wound mending, upgraded strength of the thyroid organ, diminished joint agony and improved joint pain manifestations.

To completely exploit these advantages, it's essential to pick a gadget that conveys ideal wavelengths of light. The best wavelengths of red light are in the scopes of 630-670 and 810-880.

I have the Joovv™ Light unique size with the combo Red/NIR lights. The combo light works at a wavelength of 660nm/850nm. My solitary lament isn't getting the biggest one!

This kind of treatment gives profound mending; give yourself an opportunity to encounter its advantages. I utilize mine consistently, day by day when I can. What's more, I go for 20 minutes each morning, albeit now and then I can just get 10 minutes in. I began to see a huge distinction in my skin following half a month of every day use. I began resting better and seeing improved state of mind following several months of ordinary use.

Putting resources into The Joovv™ Light is probably the best thing I've accomplished for my wellbeing as of late. On the off chance that you have any inquiries, leave them beneath!

If it's not too much trouble note that the Joovv™ Light accompanies a 2-year guarantee and a 60 Day merchandise exchange!

PAID ENDORSEMENT DISCLOSURE: In request for me to help my blogging exercises, I may get money related pay or different kinds of compensation for my underwriting, suggestion, tribute as well as connect to any items or administrations from this blog. I just prescribe items that I wholeheartedly accept to be important or that I use myself. Rubies and Radishes is a member in the Amazon Services LLC Associates Program, a subsidiary promoting program intended to give a way to locales to win publicizing charges by publicizing and connecting to amazon.com

THE BENEFITS OF THE RED AND NEAR INFRA-RED-LIGHT THERAPY

Red and close infra-red-light treatment has noteworthy potential in the recuperating procedure of our skin and bodies on an atomic level and past . This treatment is valuable in treating wounds, for example, consumes, tainted wounds, and removal wounds to guarantee a higher achievement rate for mending.

The red light invigorates the working of fibroblast,

which is answerable for the creation of collagen. At the point when fibroblast are presented to red light or approach infra-red, they make more collagen. Collagen makes up the greater part of the protein found in the human skin, the nearness of enough collagen in the body anticipate wrinkles, stretch lines, and other skin imperfections, making them less recognizable .

THE BENEFITS OF JOOVV GO RED LIGHT THERAPY

Numerous people have picked to utilize the Joovv go light treatment gadget on the grounds that the gadget has the correct blend of red-light wavelengths that can ensure further infiltration of the higher wavelength and the cell charging of the lower unmistakable range.

It is likewise long enough to cover an enormous surface territory of the body. Joovv red light treatment has a few medical advantages, which incorporate yet not restricted to:

Collagen and Anti-Aging: Joovv red light treatment feels so reviving on the grounds that it animates the creation of collagen, which gives skin its flexibility, makes the hair more grounded and enables the connective tissues to fortify its capacity to hold everything together. A few preliminaries and studies have indicated that Joovv red light treatment improves skin tone and appearance, decreases indications of maturing, and speeds the mending wounds.

Blurring scars and stretch imprints: As wonderful as parenthood may be, pregnancy stretch imprint is one lingering impact of labor. With traditional medications, it takes more time to blur off, however with the Joovv go red light, it is amazing that the imprints can blur quicker.

Expanded drive: a few bits of research has certified that red light treatment builds testosterone level and increment blood stream, prompting an expansion in moxie inside only minutes.

Decreased irritation and joint torment: one of the essential reactions to Joovv red light treatment is an articulated decrease in aggravation and oxidative worry, with fundamentally brought down joint torment.

Expanded melatonin and rest: many individuals are presented to a great deal of undesirable counterfeit light that disturbs their circadian cadence and makes it harder to rest. Joovv go red light does the inverse and helps increment the melatonin level in the body, making it simpler to nod off.

Upgraded cell flagging: Joovv go red light has a particular wavelength of light that makes a superior oxidative condition in the human body cells. This outcome in the actuation of various intracellular flagging pathways, expanded protein amalgamation, chemical enactment that keeps the body working at an ideal level.

Need to see which gadget may be directly for you? Snap Here to see the Joovv Go Device and use rebate code FATFORWEIGHTLOSS for your exceptional offer.

While the gadget has been appeared to evoke numerous valuable consequences for the human body, the above data is proposed to educate any inquiries you may have about red light and approach infrared light treatment yet doesn't supplant any medicinal counsel. In the event that you have any inquiries regarding whether this sort of treatment is appropriate for you, it is in every case best to address your PCP.

Advantages OF RED LIGHT THERAPY

Presently we should discuss a portion of the advantages

of red light treatment past simply surface level skin issues and maturing. It truly works — simply type in "when red light treatment", "red light treatment surveys" or "red light treatment tributes" into google and you'll see many stories and pictures from genuine individuals who discovered wellbeing and mending with the fuse of red light treatment into their everyday practice.

A portion OF THE HEALTH BENEFITS OF RED LIGHT THERAPY INCLUDE:

- Supports solid skin and against maturing endeavors
- Advances fat misfortune
- Helps with muscle recuperation
- Lifts state of mind and lessens pressure
- Advances hair development
- Assists with S.A.D (Seasonal Affective Disorder)
- Advances testosterone generation in men
- Advances hormone balance in ladies
- Reduces joint agony and solidness
- Reduces scarce differences and wrinkles
- Supports rest streamlining
- Counteracts repeating mouth blisters

- Advances wound recuperating
- Helps blur old scars and stretch imprints
- Aids mind wellbeing, intellectual capacity, memory, and learning
- Fixes sun harm
- Oxygenation of tissues
- Expands flow
- Advances unwinding
- Supports sound thyroid capacity
- Neutralizes the negative impacts of blue light
- Advances cell vitality
- Helps in recuperation from horrible mind wounds
- Diminishes aggravation
- Rates recuperation from preparing and thus increments physical execution
- Directs Circadian Rhythm
- Advantages patients with Alzheimer's and Dementia
- Advances collagen creation

Enlightening How Red Light Therapy Works

RLT does something amazing by conveying protected, concentrated wavelengths of regular light into your skin (up to 10 profound millimeters, to be precise) where it's consumed by your cells. This "animates the creation of collagen, elastin, and fibroblasts," says Rhonda Klein, M.D., a board-guaranteed dermatologist in Connecticut. That thus upgrades a bit of something known as ATP, the wellspring of vitality for each phone in the body (read: common vitality sans a 3:00 P.M. caffeine crash). "RLT likewise helps dissemination, carrying more oxygen and supplements to your cells and tissues," Dr. Klein says.

Interpretation? At the point when your phones are hit with the red light wavelengths, a large group of regenerative impacts happen, prompting potential advantages like more youthful looking skin, upgraded muscle fix, and decreased scarring.

As proof for RLT's advantages mounts, so do approaches to absorb them. Proficient health recognizes—your dermatologist's office, neighborhood spa, or possibly an extravagant rec center—offer an assortment of alternatives, from full-body boards that enable you to lounge in the shine to littler gadgets for more focused on medicines. You can likewise do DIY medications at home with a handheld gadget, red light face veil, or even a RLT bed, on the off chance that you need to bet everything.

Promotion

It's an extraordinary red light that conveys this exhibition upgrading support, notwithstanding; two wavelengths of red light specifically—660 nanometers and 850 nanometers—convey the best organic reaction, clarifies Michael Hamblin, M.D., a partner teacher at Harvard Medical School. The previous, 660 nanometers, is all the more immediately consumed by the skin, making it the go-to for restorative medicines, while 850 nanometer wavelengths enter further into your body to help with muscle recuperation, joint torment, and full body wellbeing.

At the end of the day, you can't simply pop a red light into your work area light and hope to kick off a cell time machine. At the point when you visit an expert, you can expect a treatment using one of these ideal wavelengths, yet on the off chance that you purchase a DIY gadget, make certain to watch that it indicates a yield force. "With such huge numbers of gadgets turning out on the web, it's a smart thought to counsel a dermatologist or other healthy skin master to control you on the best decision," says Dr. Klein. (You ought to likewise be careful about tanning salons that swap out UV bulbs for red bulbs in tanning beds and charge them as "antiaging" medications, she includes.)

Where red light becomes questionable is what number of beams you really need to absorb to get results—scientists haven't yet nailed down the ideal portion. What they can be sure of is that there isn't a dread of trying too hard. "You could utilize RLT for 24 hours as day and wouldn't harm the skin," says Dr. Hamblin. "It's practically difficult to bring on any damage."

Advantages of Red Light Therapy

Wound mending

Wolverine-esque injury mending is only one of the numerous advantages touted by advocates of RLT—and there's no deficiency of research to affirm it truly helps you recuperate quicker. A recent report discovered red light treatment advanced "expanded tissue fix and recuperating... [plus] useful impacts on wrinkles, skin break out scars, hypertrophic scars, and mending of copies."

Muscle fix and recuperation

With regards to muscle fix and recuperation, proof recommend RLT has benefits when utilized both pre- and postworkout. A recent report found that the restorative method prompted diminished muscle quality misfortune, less muscle irritation, and less scope of-movement weaknesses for as long as four days after exercise. A later 2018 examination likewise demonstrated that RLT both when exercise decreases knee muscle weariness.

Help with discomfort

At the center of a considerable lot of these advantages is RLT's capability to decrease aggravation and agony. Scientists have discovered that RLT presentation can help decrease torment for osteoarthritis knee torment, meniscus tears, general knee torment, rheumatoid joint pain, and back torment. The information on red light treatment for relief from discomfort is so persuading the FDA has endorsed it as a treatment for treating minor torments and joint pain.

Skin issues

One of the most mainstream employments of RLT is to clear up skin issues like skin break out. "I wouldn't customarily suggest red light treatment for serious skin inflammation, yet it's a magnificent added substance treatment that is sheltered and well-endured by all skin types and tones," says Angela Lamb, M.D., partner educator of the division of dermatology at the Icahn School of Medicine at Mount Sinai Hospital in New York City. The skin-clearing mystery lies in RLT's mitigating impacts, says Dr. Klein. It likewise helps normally decline oil generation and bacterial levels in your skin—no drying impacts or unforgiving synthetic compounds required.

Red light skin break out medicines are genuinely simple to discover—most dermatologists offer them in-office or you can purchase an at-home gadget. Dr. Sheep suggests LightStim for Acne ($165). Dr. Klein enjoys Neutrogena's Light Therapy Acne Mask ($35) for at-home use.

While there's strong proof that RLT benefits skin break out, the examination is as yet inadequate with regards to with regards to psoriasis. "Right now, psoriasis most likely has minimal measure of information with regards to red light treatment alone being a compelling treatment," says Dr. Klein.

Antiaging

Alright, so what about that entire wellspring of-youth thing? There are a lot of concentrates to help RLT's antiaging ability, for example, a recent report which discovered that clients of RLT experienced altogether improved skin appearance and an expansion in collagen. "Science shows that red light treatment ensures existing collagen and lifts new generation," says Dr. Sheep. "Additionally it assists with surface, tone, pore size, and wrinkles."

The Verdict

So is RLT extremely enchantment? Not exactly—no treatment can give you Wolverine-like powers at this time. Be that as it may, the science behind red light treatment is unimaginably encouraging. "Practically, you can expect RLT to improve your skin's tone and surface," Dr. Klein says. "We realize that it alleviates aggravation, improves gentle skin inflammation, and proactively treats barely recognizable differences and wrinkles, notwithstanding different advantages."

The jury is still out with respect to the definite measurements required for an ideal impact, yet meanwhile, you can breathe a sigh of relief knowing there's demonstrated antiaging benefits and no destructive reactions.

The Benefits for Your Skin

- Red light treatment makes a solid shine about your face
- smooths in general skin tone
- constructs collagen, diminishing wrinkles, including crow's feet, under eye wrinkles, brow wrinkles and giggle lines
- speeds the mending of imperfections, similar to skin inflammation and rosacea
- fixes sun harm
- decreases redness, flushing, and broken vessels
- blurs scars and stretch imprints
- carries more dampness to your skin
- forestalls male pattern baldness and animates regrowth
- treats a developing rundown of skin conditions

Red Light Therapy for Skin Rejuvenation

Red light effectively infiltrates the skin, supports flow and carrying more blood and supplements to the territory. It additionally animates crucial collagen and elastin creation. Collagen helps full the skin, while elastin firms the skin. The red light is empowering and fixing harmed cells, animating collagen and elastin and giving the skin back its energetic look.

Home gadgets for skin restoration ordinarily utilize obvious red light at a wavelength of 660nm – That enters tissue to a profundity of around 8-10 mm – Making it progressively helpful for treating issues near the outside of the skin, for example,

1. Wrinkles and scarce differences

2. Fixing and firming (non-careful cosmetic touch up elective,)

3. Imperfections and redness

4. Hostile to maturing

5. Age spots and hyperpigmentation on face, hands, neck

6. Skin inflammation scars

Red Light Therapy for Skin Problems

As I composed above, red light advances the mending of the skin thus can be utilized adequately for some skin issues, without prescription (we as a whole know their risky reactions), and synthetic stacked salves and creams. You can utilize a home gadget for these conditions (Warning: Do not utilize it on the off chance that you have a functioning skin disease):

1. Consumes

2. Skin break out Scars

3. Rosacea

4. Skin inflammation

5. Psoriasis

6. Competitor's foot

Red Light Therapy for Pain Relief

Red light treatment for relief from discomfort is a delicate, non-intrusive, sedate free, and synthetic free elective that has been appeared to decrease and now and again even dispense with a throbbing painfulness. From the start it sounds strange. In what manner can light help with my incessant back torment? All things considered, it's very straightforward. The infrared light (imperceptible light) infiltrates further in our body and fixes or recovers cell parts. The infrared light likewise enacts the creation of endorphins and squares torment transmitting synthetic substances. The home gadgets for this reason regularly utilize Infrared light (profound infiltrating light) – at 880nm, which enters to a profundity of around 30-40 mm, making it a compelling relief from discomfort for:

1. Herniated and protruding circles

2. Muscle related back agony

3. Osteoarthritis

4. Fibromyalgia

5. Pulled and stressed muscles, Muscle fits

6. Irritation

7. Nerve wounds

8. Sports wounds: bone breaks and chips, sprains, tennis

elbow and so forth.

9. Neck agony and solidness

Is There a Device That Combines Red and Infrared Lights In One?

Indeed, the top red light treatment home gadgets consolidate both noticeable red lights and infrared lights so you can utilize them for BOTH skin restoration and relief from discomfort.

These top of the line gadgets are: DPL Deep Penetrating Light Therapy (My undisputed top choice), Baby Quasar Red Light Therapy Device, Omnilux MD – New U and LightStim.

What are the Benefits of Red Light Therapy?

Here are the accompanying advantages of Red Light Therapy announced in peer checked on medicinal diaries.

The medications with the utilization of Red Light Therapy that have been affirmed by the FDA incorporate relief from discomfort including torment from joint pain, Anti-maturing, skin inflammation treatment, male pattern baldness and regrowth, fat misfortune.

It ought to be noticed that the treatment isn't endorsed, rather the gadget. The endorsement or FDA leeway implies that the gadget is sheltered to utilize and that it works.

Along these lines, generally, since the treatment is endorsed, the more significant inquiry is the gadget FDA cleared or FDA affirmed.

Extra advantages of red light treatment that have been accounted for in restorative diaries or individuals have found are recorded beneath. In certain occasions, the advantages recorded beneath have been seen in pet lab mice or guinea pigs. Despite the fact that there are not yet human investigations for specific medications, there are narrative proof that they additionally deal with people the equivalent.

Blood

Lifts glutathione: our bodies ace cancer prevention agent, ace invulnerability and ace detoxifier

Expands blood stream

Decreases Inflammation in skin and some more profound tissues

Vitality

Improves vitality

Head/Mental

Decreases cerebral pains, sinus agony and weight, nasal blockage, sore throats, ear throbs

Give help of hacking

Decreases strain and tension

Decreases crabbiness

Muscles and Joints

Stops muscle fits and decreases events

Decreases joint firmness by as much as 20%

Decrease torment and growing when applied over the skin, muscles, and joint torment

Diminishes torment

Knee torment decrease

Back agony decrease

Neck torment decrease

Post surgeries improvement

Careful injury torment decrease

what's more, abbreviated careful recuperating times

Sciatica torment decrease

Piriformis torment decrease

Joint pain torment decrease

Joint pain irritation decrease

Broken bones recuperating time diminished (expands osteoblasts or new bone cells)

Carpal passage disorder alleviation

Fibromyalgia help with discomfort

Foot torment (plantar fasciitis) help

Shoulder relief from discomfort

Sprains recuperate quicker

Torn tendons recuperating time abbreviated

Tendonitis help

Nerve Regeneration

Can advance nerve recovery

Skin

Carries an energetic solid gleam to your face

Advances solid skin

Advances smooths skin tone

. Improves flexibility of collagen filaments

Builds collagen

Decreases wrinkles, crow's feet, eye wrinkles, temple wrinkles and giggle lines

Mends imperfections, skin break out and rosacea

Enables wounding to vanish

Fixes skin harm from the sun

Decreases redness, flushing, and broken vessels

Blurs scars and stretch imprints

Builds dampness to your skin (when utilized with Water Cures Protocol)

Eases back and even stops male pattern baldness and invigorates hair development

Skin conditions it can improve are constantly developing

Recuperates bug nibbles

Recuperates minor consumes

Mends cuts and scratches

Assists fix with drying sSkin (when utilizing the Water Cures Protocol)

Diminishes flushing

Scars and Stretch Marks

Causes scar keloids to vanish

Causes stretch imprints to vanish

Rest

Diminishes time taken to nod off

Empowers further, progressively tranquil rest

Teeth and Gums

Regrow bones around teeth

Reestablishes gum wellbeing

Improve dental wellbeing

Spare free teeth, fixing them in their attachment

Wounds

Accelerates twisted mending to days, not weeks

Rates twisted Healing in ineffectively

recuperating wounds

Reestablishes or improves scope of movement

Diminishes irritation and joint torment

Extra Benefits

Burrowed free

No synthetic substances

Non-obtrusive (no needles, cutting or consuming)

No torment (doesn't tingle, consume or sting)

No personal time or recuperation time from treatment

Alright for a wide range of skin

no symptoms, either short or long haul

Can act naturally regulated once prepared

How Often/How Long Do I Need To Be Treated?

There are various contemplations to decide how regularly and to what extent you should be blessed to receive get the best advantages of Red Light Therapy.

Liquid, Electrolytes and the Benefits of Red Light Therapy

While there are few individuals who will get restricted outcomes (most advisors have a 90% achievement rate. As far as we can tell, while consolidating the Water Cures Protocol, we have had a 98% achievement rate to-date settling the conditions RLT is affirmed for. The explanation is straightforward, our cells can work best when hydrated and work ineffectively when they are either got dried out or lacking appropriate electrolyte balance.

One factor to help decide how well it will function for you includes to what degree you utilize different modalities, for example, diet, hydration and common topical operators to improve your wellbeing preceding adding the Red Light Therapy to what you are doing.

How Often: You can have medications as frequently as like clockwork. This is the most that individuals who buy the lights and self treat ought to do.

Be that as it may, a great many people just get treatment from prepared Energy Light Therapists from at regular intervals to once per week. A few conditions require extra presentation or dosages. Most medicines will require week after week medications for as long as five weeks and once the advantages of red light treatment have been accomplished, as meager as once a month insofar as diet and hydration are thought about.

A few conditions won't require any further portions once an ideal outcome has been accomplished. Others, for example, horrendous mind damage may require day by day use for a considerable length of time, years or in any event, for a lifetime. In such cases, it is an exchange off, have improved existence with every day medications or a less quality life and no medicines. Such conditions will require owning the gadget to make day by day utilize conceivable.

To what extent for Treatments: Light introduction time is an inquiry concerning what might be viewed as the portion. It includes the length or number of minutes you need presentation to the lights. It is comparative with how near the influenced territory the lights are, at the end of the day, how near the skin the light is. The more remote away, the less portion that is gotten. On account of close to infrared, the diodes should contact if not as close as conceivable to get the best advantage.

A treatment can be cultivated in as not many as two or three minutes or may take as long as 45 minutes and may utilize a mix of frequencies and heartbeats.

Once more, this will rely upon what advantages of red light treatment are being looked for. It will likewise rely upon the extra dietary contemplations you incorporate. At long last, it will rely upon your body and your skin. Everybody will be extraordinary.

Additionally it ought to be noted, for those utilizing the gadget all alone, on the off chance that you utilize the gadget excessively long or not long enough, it won't work. The gadgets you buy ought to have a worked in clock so that once the ideal measure of time they are applied is come to, they will be naturally killed.

We spread this data in our Red Light Therapy Guide which comes free with any red light item you buy from us. Moreover, instructing is incorporated with the buy. On the off chance that you read online surveys, you may discover numerous who will say that the gadgets don't work. While their remarks might be valid as to their experience, it could be because of abuse or absence of sufficient information on how they work.

Hence, we like to have an individual really get a treatment by a prepared Light Energy Therapist preceding buying any item with the goal that they can completely and effectively experience the item and how well it functions.

On the off chance that you as of now have a red light treatment gadget, you can buy the guide so as to figure out how to more readily utilize your gadget.

While many get brings about the principal treatment, a few conditions require extra medications, even numerous for a little while. A few conditions require three times each week and may take a month prior emotional enhancements are noted. On account of nerve recovery, a while of day by day use might be required, making owning your own gadget or even a framework progressively affordable.

At times, the medicines might be required forever. This was the end on the effective utilization of Red Light Therapy on horrendous cerebrum damage patients. In the two cases in the clinical path, the advantages of red light treatment was acknowledged both just after the damage and quite a while after the damage. In the two cases, every day utilize was required. Along these lines, owning a framework will make the procedure simpler and increasingly reasonable.

Extra factors incorporate age, state of skin, diet, generally wellbeing, sicknesses you are distressed with and particularly any prescriptions you are utilizing.

Symptoms: In the a great many research papers distributed on the advantages of red light treatment, there have been no detailed reactions. Nonetheless, there are episodic revealing of what some have encountered. This could be because of inappropriate use (counting ill-advised preparing) and ill-advised introduction times.

Security: While thought about safe, there are conceivable negative and even a potential damage that can emerge out of the utilization of particular sorts of Red Light Therapy. Contingent upon whether you are on meds, have certain medical problems or are simply touchy, you may encounter cerebral pains, eye strain, fractiousness, rest unsettling influences and a sleeping disorder.

While one of the advantages of red light treatment is advancing rest, blue light treatment may obstruct rest.

These potential negatives are not found in the exploration, rather have been accounted for narratively. While the red lights can be utilized on the eyes, this should just be finished by an advisor who is prepared for utilizing them on the eyes or an eye specialist prepared in RLT.

Those with epilepsy should utilize the RLT with alert, particularly with the beating lights.

The visual unsettling influences are gentle and leave rapidly. While these are referenced in writing, in my training, none of those I have worked so far have encountered any of these impacts. I don't do chip away at the eyes, along these lines no visual unsettling influence has been experienced. One individual reaction I have actually encountered, my sight has improved without glasses.

Utilize Extra Caution If:

In the event that you have an illness of the eye that include the retina (diabetes) or use photosensitizing drugs, for example, lithium, phenothiazine antipsychotics, melatonin, or on the off chance that you are on anti-infection agents that have a symptom of causing photograph affectability.

In the event that you have skin malignant growth or foundational lupus erythematosus you ought not utilize RLT except if treated by an accomplished advisor. Particularly you ought not utilize full range light and on the off chance that you do, it should just be done under the supervision of an accomplished MD.

In the event that you are obtaining a gadget for individual use, it is basic that you be watchful with respect to any adjustments in your status in regards to the above concerns. Medicinal services experts who are prepared in the utilization of light vitality treatment or photobiomodulation realize the worries identified with non-ionizing radiation delivered by the light-emanating gadget just as the potential harmful synthetic perils that can result from introduction to photosensitizing specialists.

You ought to have and utilize eye assurance when utilizing red light treatment of any sort and particularly the LLLT or low level laser treatment. Also, if treating wounds, you should comprehend the mending procedure and pursue the conventions of where to uncover and where and what some portion of the injury to shield from the ionizing radiation of the lights for ideal advantages of red light treatment.

Opposite Side-impacts of Light Therapy

While light treatment just uses the frequencies found in

noticeable light and no negative reactions have been accounted for in writing, alert still should be worked out. The individuals who experience non-occasional sorrow may encounter craziness. Since we have seen and have gotten various reports of melancholy being wiped out with the Water Cures Protocol (which produces glutathione) and by expanding glutathione through the eating regimen, for some, this hazard might be wiped out with diet and hydration. On the off chance that fundamental in any case, basically lessen or stop the utilization of the red light treatment until steady and afterward continue so as to get the full advantages of red light treatment.

With certain shades of light, for example, green, there is an expanded potential hazard for skin malignant growth advancement sometime down the road.

It has been proposed that eye strain and impermanent migraines caused might be brought about by the light. There is no signs that this causes lasting damage.

As of now, we need more research accessible for utilizing it to treat malignant growth. Therefor, we don't prescribe RLT for malignant growth right now. Be that as it may, there is promising examination thinking about this probability.

The History of Red Therapy Light Use

Red light treatment has obtained a lifetime of experience already. In 1903 doctor Niels Ryberg Finsen won the Nobel Prize in Medicine for his effective treatment of smallpox and lupus with red light. Russia utilizes low level laser treatment in their standard medicinal consideration (and they have since the 1970s). The Russians additionally distributed several investigations throughout the decades on the advantages of red treatment light. Shockingly, not many of these investigations have been converted into English.

Red light treatment has generally been disregarded by the US and western Europe up to this point. Anyway it's been utilized in a clinical setting since the 1980s in Japan, China, Canada, Northern Ireland, Vietnam, Latin America, and Eastern Europe.

The Benefits of Red Therapy Light

Despite the fact that the western world is out of date with red treatment light, solid proof backings its medical advantages. It is FDA endorsed for interminable joint agony, slow to mend wounds, wrinkles, male pattern baldness and skin break out. Numerous others have utilized it effectively for different issues, similar to psoriasis, improved dissemination and better invulnerable capacity.

Here's an incomplete rundown of the proof based employments of red treatment light:

It revives facial skin and smooths skin tone.

Red light forms collagen in the skin to lessen wrinkles.

It fixes sun harm.

Red light actuates the lymphatic framework for conceivably improved detoxification.

Diminishes irritation in the skin.

Helps blur scars and stretch imprints.

Improves hair development to turn around going bald.

Animates moderate mending wounds.

Can counteract repeating mouth blisters, or herpes simplex.

Supportive in the present moment for carpal passage disorder.

Gainful for skin to diminish dermatitis, rosacea, and skin break out.

1. Better Circulation and Collagen Production

At the point when the light enters through the epidermal and dermal skin layers, it expands flow to help structure new vessels. It likewise expands collagen generation and fibroblasts. While topically applied collagen is pointless, I every now and again devour it for the strength of my nails, skin, hair, and joints. Red treatment light improves collagen levels normally by setting off the body to deliver its very own greater amount. Since collagen involves about 70% of the protein in our skin, it's a serious deal!

Expanded collagen doesn't simply give the skin a sans wrinkle shine, however its capacity to improve joint wellbeing makes it incredible for joint pain sufferers. It tends to be useful for those with an assortment of agonizing musculoskeletal issues. The expanded flow and calming impacts that red treatment light gives likewise help decrease torment and recuperate the body.

2. Twisted Healing with Red Light Therapy

Fibroblasts in our skin orchestrate collagen, keep up connective tissue and are vital to wound mending. Red treatment light animates fibroblasts to carry out their responsibility, and builds flow for quicker twisted fix time. Individuals have additionally utilized this treatment for consumes, removal wounds, skin unites and tainted injuries. It's been effectively utilized for skin harm brought about by malignant growth medications, incorporating those in the mouth and bodily fluid layers.

In a recent report, specialists found that red light treatment fundamentally improved colitis side effects in mice. The light treatment supported in their mucosal mending. Dental specialists have additionally effectively utilized red treatment lights to recuperate bruises and scraped areas in the bodily fluid films of the mouth. It's additionally been found to counteract repeating mouth blisters that happen along the mouth.

3. A Remedy for Hair Loss

I have a lot of common cures on my site for how to improve hair development, however red light treatment might be another approach to turn around thinning up top. A 24-week study exhibited that red treatment light fundamentally improved hair thickness and hair thickness with no genuine responses. Members wore a head protector that radiated red treatment light to accomplish this impact, however I've discovered that greater gadgets (like this one) are simpler to utilize and profit the remainder of the body too.

4. Recuperate Faster from Injury and Illness

Red light treatment builds course and ATP creation all through the body which may help speed recuperating during times of sickness. It likewise invigorates lymph framework action and phagocytosis, the procedure of cells cleaning house.

Albeit red treatment light adjusts the resistant framework, a recent report with mice found that over treatment really brought about safe concealment. Since not a great deal of research has been done here, it's indistinct exactly how advantageous it is for the safe framework.

5. Help for the Thyroid

One of the central reasons I began investigating red light

treatment is a result of the potential for improved thyroid capacity. There are a few convincing investigations that take a gander at the advantages of red light and approach infrared treatment for thyroid wellbeing. As somebody who has battled with Hashimoto's Thyroiditis, I was keen on attempting this sort of treatment.

One randomized, fake treatment controlled clinical examination from 2013 took a gander at the advantages of light treatment on interminable immune system thyroiditis. This investigation indicated a general improvement in thyroid wellbeing from close to infrared and light treatment. Numerous members had the option to diminish or dispense with their thyroid drug. Actually, an alarming 47 percent of the members never again required medicine during the whole nine-month follow-up after the light treatment. This is stunning as a great many people are informed that they will require thyroid medicine for the remainder of their lives.

When taking a gander at Hashimoto's (immune system thyroid issues) explicitly, the investigation found a decrease in thyroid peroxidase (TPOAb) antibodies. These antibodies show the nearness of an immune system thyroid condition.

Different investigations have appeared:

a recent report from Russia found that red light treatment helped 38% of members diminish thyroid prescription dose (17% halted medicine totally)

A recent report on postsurgical thyroid patients found that red light treatment diminished the requirement for drug by up to 75%

I for one began looking into this advantage in the wake of seeing specialists utilize this treatment for thyroid infection while visiting a characteristic medication center in Switzerland. While I was there, they had me wear a red light treatment gadget on my neck to profit my thyroid. I've been proceeding with this treatment at home with my red light.

6. A Promising Therapy for Psoriasis

A little scale study distributed in the diary of Photomedicine and Laser Surgery discovered advantages for psoriasis sufferers. Skin plaques improved by 60-100% when treated with both red treatment light and infrared light, similar to that utilized in a sauna. The infrared light quieted aggravation, while the shorter red wavelengths recuperated the skin's surface.

Despite the fact that I don't have psoriasis, I've actually seen skin profits by utilizing a mix light (I have the Joovv combo unit connected beneath) that consolidates close infrared ranges (810-880) and noticeable red ranges (630-670).

7. Help for Acne, Rosacea, and Eczema

The collagen and ATP invigorating advantages of red light treatment make it a promising answer for skin issues like skin break out, rosacea, and dermatitis. By and by, the primary advantages I saw were in lessening stretch checks and wrinkles. After some time, I've additionally seen new hair development on my hairline.

The most effective method to Use a Red Therapy Light

A few spas, rheumatologists, and dermatologists offer red light treatment medications. A specialist may likewise have the option to give a referral to a prepared proficient. Since there are just a couple of FDA affirmed utilizes for red treatment light, treatment may not be canvassed by protection now and again.

There are likewise salons and spas that offer red light treatment. These choices regularly extend from $50-100 a session.

I've discovered that it is increasingly advantageous (and likely a lot less expensive) to get the advantages of red light treatment at home.

There are a lot of at home gadgets available to be purchased from an assortment of producers. I needed to discover a gadget that utilized a blend of wavelengths for most extreme advantage. Thusly, I would get the advantage of the more profound infiltration of the higher wavelength and the cell "charging" of the lower unmistakable range. Two extraordinary decisions are the Joovv light or Red Therapy Company light. I've attempted both and discover them similar.

Medical advantages OF RED LIGHT THERAPY

Taking a gander at the rundown beneath, it appears that red light treatment resembles enchantment.

As Ari Whitten says, "If there were a medication that had logical research indicating every one of these advantages, it would be an outright blockbuster sedate for pharmaceutical organizations it would be hailed as a 'supernatural occurrence medication' and endorsed to fundamentally everybody. Here's the best part: That 'sedate" exists. It's only not as a pill. It's as NIR and red light treatment!"

Here goes–red and NIR light treatment has been appeared to:

Diminish interminable irritation (model investigation)

Improves insusceptible framework (model examination)

Manufacture flexibility to worry at the cell level (source)

Battle some immune system conditions and improves thyroid capacity (model investigation: decrease in Hashimoto's TPO antibodies by 39% and measurement of thyroid substitution medicine)

Improve hormonal wellbeing (for instance, by reestablishing the liver, significant for your thyroid and estrogen)

Streamline your mind and psychological capacity; expands neuroprotection

Improves state of mind, despondency, and uneasiness (model investigation)

Increment richness

Defeat weariness and improve vitality levels, and assists with rest (model examination)

Battle the oxidative harm that drives maturing

Reduction torment (model here for low back agony, constant torment, joint torment, and fibromyalgia)

Increment quality, perseverance, and bulk; expands collagen creation

Accelerate wound/damage recuperating

Battle skin maturing, wrinkles, hyperpigmentation, skin conditions, and cellulite Lose fat (almost twice likewise with diet and exercise alone) (model investigation)

Helps hair regrowth

Recovers immature microorganisms (model examination)

I realize it truly seems 'unrealistic', be that as it may, given there are more than 3,000 companion audited logical investigations on this innovation, there's unquestionably something to it! Presently, more research is as yet expected to see every one of the subtleties and best applications, be that as it may, it's time we start discussing red light treatment as a genuine mending methodology.

Likewise, it's imperative to note here that these advantages are not generally observed with only a solitary session (or even a couple of sessions), yet rather when rehashed after some time.

In case you're as yet distrustful, think about this: what do we do to think about new children, specific creatures? We put them under a red light warmth light (hatchery). Shouldn't something be said about when infants have jaundice? The doc puts them under a bili-light, a type of phototherapy. On the off chance that you have psoriasis, your dermatologist may have prescribed bright light phototherapy. Light treatment works!

Diminish wrinkles and indications of maturing by invigorating collagen development. Red light advances the generation of collagen, which is liable for keeping your skin flexible and firm. Use RLT two times every day for 10 minutes to smooth out barely recognizable differences and wrinkles on your face.

Utilizing RLT on the skin of your face will likewise smooth out the surface of your skin and lessen the size of your pores after some time.

New collagen cells set aside a long effort to develop. Try not to hope to see hostile to maturing results until following 3 months of consistent RLT.

Calm skin break out by improving dissemination and diminishing expanding. RLT improves dissemination and decreases aggravation any place it's applied. At the point when utilized on skin break out, this outcomes in especially terrible flaws getting less excruciating and the lymphatic framework being better ready to clean up waste.

For treating skin inflammation, lower dosages of red light are best. Instead of over-burdening your face at the same time, embrace a "little and frequently" RLT schedule. Apply red light to skin break out spots two times per day for 3 minutes each time and keep up this routine for about fourteen days to get results.

Blue light treatment is great at murdering specific sorts of skin break out causing microorganisms. Think about utilizing the two types of light treatment simultaneously to both lessen and forestall skin inflammation breakouts.

Picture titled Benefit from Red Light Therapy

Treat normal skin conditions like dermatitis and psoriasis. The calming properties of RLT have helped numerous individuals get alleviation from the distress of aggravation brought about by skin conditions. Use RLT to diminish the tingling and uneasiness brought about by conditions like skin inflammation and psoriasis.

RLT medicines for psoriasis have not been completely looked into enough to make items be promoted explicitly for that reason. Be that as it may, RLT gadgets utilized for against maturing and agony medicines can for the most part additionally be utilized for psoriasis.

You may have more achievement treating psoriasis by joining RLT with close to infrared light.

Anticipate male pattern baldness and invigorate development. RLT has been appeared at times to animate hair follicle development, in this manner halting and turning around male pattern baldness in the two people. In spite of the fact that investigations of this utilization of RLT have delivered blended outcomes, there's great narrative proof for its utilization as a male pattern baldness remedy.

RLT medications to counteract balding ought to be controlled 2-3 times every week, for 8-15 minutes every session. These can be done at an uncommon RLT hair salon or at home.

Utilizing RLT to treat balding requires a great deal of time and duty. Try not to hope to see positive outcomes sooner than 12 weeks.

Fix regular corrective harm to your skin. The most well known utilization of RLT is as a skin rejuvenator and repairer. Past treating constant skin conditions and significant harms, RLT can likewise be utilized to treat ordinary imperfections like cuts and scratches and the scars they depart behind.

Utilizing RLT as a component of your emergency treatment for minor cuts and scratches can help make these wounds less excruciating and accelerate the recuperating procedure.

Scars, either from cuts or from skin break out, can be altogether diminished after some time through normal introduction to red light, because of the effect RLT has on the skin's capacity to mend.

Make your skin more beneficial through improved narrow development. RLT expands course and prompts the expanded arrangement of vessels in the influenced region. Vessels help carry oxygen and supplements to skin cells, thus more vessels will help make your skin look a lot more beneficial and more youthful.

This will likewise smooth your general skin tone and give your face an overflowing gleam.

RLT likewise improves the wellbeing of your skin by expanding lymph framework action, which lessens growing and puffiness accordingly.

Treating Wounds and Pain with RLT

Diminish joint solidness and agony. RLT is thought to have comparative impacts as warmth when applied to solid or agonizing joints; that is, it can help decrease joint torment by as much as 20%. Use RLT related to active recuperation to help ease joint agony and diminish solidness over time.

Joints can get stuck in an agony cycle, in which joints

hurt and turn out to be solid, driving you to utilize them less, prompting expanded torment and solidness because of absence of utilization. Utilizing RLT can help decrease solidness enough to empower you to utilize your joints all the more uninhibitedly and along these lines break out of this agony cycle.

With regards to treating joint agony, make a point to utilize RLT related to non-intrusive treatment. RLT without anyone else's input won't be sufficient to fix joint torment.

Accelerate the mending of wounds. Red light can enable an injury to mend up to 200% quicker than expected. Use RLT as a component of medical aid and post-medical procedure twisted medications to enable your body to mend its injuries more quickly.

For a formerly non-shutting wound, it will take approximately 4 two months of ceaseless RLT treatment to completely close the injury, contingent upon the conditions.

Notwithstanding advancing collagen and fine development, RLT likewise animates tissue granulation, which includes the arrangement of new connective tissue over the opening of wounds.

Treat the indications of Restless Leg Syndrome. A recent report found that RLT, related to approach infrared light treatment, can achieve an improvement in the indications of those experiencing Restless Leg Syndrome. Consider joining RLT into your general treatment routine on the off chance that you experience the ill effects of Restless Leg Syndrome.

Sufferers who attempted RLT saw their side effects altogether improved for up to about a month after their underlying red light treatment.

In the event that you experience the ill effects of Restless Leg Syndrome, converse with your primary care physician before depending entirely on RLT for treatment rather than progressively ordinary dopamine-influencing drugs.

Improve lower back torment and sciatica. The mitigating properties of RLT have had across the board accomplishment in easing back agony in numerous individuals. Use RLT in the event that you have back agony, neck torment, or sciatica to decrease aggravation and distress and reestablish a sound scope of motion.

For help with discomfort, it's prescribed that you use RLT on the zone two times every day for about fourteen days, at that point proceeding with 1 or 2 sessions for each week after the torment has gone down.

Make a point to utilize RLT related to exercise based recuperation for the best outcomes in treating back torment. Converse with your primary care physician to decide the best treatment plan for your particular circumstance.

Buy a gadget fit to your condition in the event that you need to do RLT at home. When acquiring a RLT gadget for at-home use, you'll need to consider both expense and capacity. Ensure the gadget you purchase has the correct characteristics for treating your particular condition.

Various conditions (e.g., joint torment, skin inflammation, wrinkles, and so on.) require various wavelengths of red light to be effectively treated with RLT. Just purchase items that are advertised to treat explicit infirmities, as these gadgets will have the correct wavelength of light.

In case you're uncertain what wavelength of light you need, look for your condition in an Internet web index alongside "LLLT" or "photobiomodulation." If inquire about has been done on treating your condition with

RLT, a prescribed wavelength will in all likelihood come up in your outcomes (e.g., 620 nm for treating most skin conditions).

You can buy a RLT gadget through an online retailer, at a dermatologist's office, or perhaps at your nearby drug store. Costs regularly extend from $100 to $300.

Visit a RLT salon on the off chance that you can't buy an at-home gadget. On the off chance that you can't gain admittance to a RLT gadget in your general vicinity, or would prefer not to stress over treating yourself effectively, visit a spa or hair salon that highlights RLT to have experts do your treatment.

Spa or salon medicines by and large cost $300 for a 75-minute session. Despite the fact that this choice is more costly than purchasing a gadget for home use, it is undeniably increasingly advantageous and unwinding.

Scanning for your zone in addition to "Red light treatment" in an Internet web crawler is a decent method to see if any neighborhood spas offer RLT sessions.

Get ready for your treatment by covering defenseless zones. RLT utilizes a splendid light that can be entirely awkward to your eyes and skin in the event that they're left uncovered. Before starting RLT all over, place defensive goggles over your eyes to sift through brilliant red light. In the event that there are portions of your body delicate to warmth or light, spread them with fabric.

It's suggested that you spread tattoos when directing RLT, as the impacts of red light on tattoos isn't completely comprehended yet.

Red light is consumed by most textures, so setting garments or wraps over your skin will be sufficient to keep red light from overcoming.

Note that in case you're utilizing RLT to accelerate the mending procedure for an injury, any gauzes on the injury should be expelled for the treatment to have any impact.

Complete RLT medications consistently or consistently as required. For RLT to be compelling, pursue a standard treatment plan dependent on your particular condition. Albeit each condition has its own suggested treatment plan, most regimens call for every day RLT for in any event 2 weeks to get huge results

Day by day RLT sessions regularly last somewhere in

the range of 3 and 10 minutes.

For long haul support take a shot at your skin or different illnesses, numerous regimens call for RLT once per week.

What are the advantages?

As referenced above, there are still a few inquiries regarding how precisely red light treatment functions, yet here are a portion of its most encouraging advantages that have been found to date:

1. It mends scars and wounds.

In the event that despite everything you have scars from your skin inflammation perplexed adolescent years, on the off chance that you've as of late experienced consumes, or on the off chance that your injuries will in general mend gradually under any conditions, at that point red light treatment might be a choice. It's idea to help skin cells work all the more effectively and fix harm by invigorating mitochondria and foundational microorganisms.

"I believe it's incredible from an expanding mitochondrial work stance," says practical medication expert and mbg Collective part Will Cole, D.C., IFMCP, who prescribes it to his patients.

Research implies that skin issues like these react better to the lower end of the red light range. In one examination, patients with mellow to direct skin break out got red light treatment in two unique wavelengths on either side of their face—630 nm on the right, 890 nm on the left—and just the lower wavelength fundamentally diminished skin inflammation sores. In another examination, patients with diabetes encountered a huge decrease in the size and agony of their diabetic foot ulcers with 12 sessions of red light treatment at 632.8 nm.

2. It advances collagen creation.

Notwithstanding its enhancing benefits, red light treatment may likewise help counter regular skin gives that happen with age, as decreased collagen generation (which starts declining around age 30), which can expand the presence of scarcely discernible differences. One examination found that patients accepting red light treatment all over two times per week for 30 all out sessions experienced improved skin composition, skin tone, skin smoothness, and collagen thickness (as estimated with a ultrasonographic test). Truth be told, the examination incorporated some when pictures, which are really amazing.

3. It advances hair development.

The most widely recognized kind of male pattern baldness, androgenetic alopecia, influences 50 percent of men over age 40 and 75 percent of ladies more than 65, and there are just two drugs affirmed to help counter it. In any case, investigate uncovers that red light treatment might be a ground-breaking, medicate free arrangement. One research survey found that red light treatment was sheltered and viable for advancing hair development in the two people. It appears to work by invigorating undifferentiated organisms in the hair follicle and moving follicles into the anagen stage (the dynamic development stage). More research is expected to decide the ideal wavelength for advancing hair development, however one examination found that ladies who got red light treatment at 650 nm each other day for 17 weeks encountered a 51 percent expansion in hair thickness.

4. It facilitates torment joint, muscle, and ligament torment.

Since red and close infrared light infiltrates further than different wavelengths, it has the one of a kind capacity to treat issues underneath the skin's surface also, similar to joint agony and muscle and ligament wounds. One of the first employments of red light treatment was in the treatment of carpal passage disorder, and research shows it can decrease torment and improve hold quality among carpal passage patients. An examination survey additionally uncovers that red light treatment is a fantastic asset in the treatment of skeletal muscle wounds because of the way that it decreases the aggravation and expands angiogenesis (the advancement of fresh recruits vessels). Furthermore, agonizing conditions like rheumatoid joint inflammation, osteoarthritis, tendinitis, plantar fasciitis, and back agony all react decidedly to red light treatment.

5. It speeds recuperation and lifts perseverance.

Red light treatment has advantages for male and female competitors, as well. One examination found that men who took an interest in extreme exercise and furthermore got red light treatment experienced improved execution and less exercise-incited muscle irritation. While another investigation on female b-ball players found that red light treatment improved perseverance just as rest. It's idea that red light treatment helps mitochondria produce vitality all the more effectively, making muscles more averse to encounter weariness.

6. Lessens symptoms of malignancy treatment.

Research directed by NASA has discovered that red light treatment enables counter a side to impact of chemotherapy called oral mucositis, portrayed by very difficult bruises, redness, dryness, and copying sensations in the mouth and throat. A two-year preliminary where malignancy patients were given a far red and close infrared LED treatment established that 96 percent of patients experienced diminished torment because of this treatment. This is extraordinary news since it could help increment nourishment admission, diminish utilization of painkillers, and lift resolve among disease patients.

What are the reactions of red light treatment?

There don't seem, by all accounts, to be many symptoms. Truth be told, some exploration papers have expressed that there is "a practically complete nonattendance of symptoms" related with red light treatment. Salazar concurs, including that it's "by and large safe for all skin types, in any event, for ladies who are pregnant." Anecdotal records uncover that a few people see red light treatment as disturbing or troublesome to the eyes, however this can be helped by wearing tanning bed goggles.

Certain red light treatment gadgets are even affirmed by the FDA to treat male pattern baldness, carpal passage disorder, muscle and joint agony, and moderate recuperating wounds. Be that as it may, distinctive wellbeing conditions have diverse ideal wavelength portions, and research proposes that lower dosages can regularly be progressively powerful. So it's significant that you locate a certified expert to oversee red light treatment fittingly for the particular condition you're attempting to treat or that you discover a FDA-affirmed gadget and adhere to the producer's guidelines cautiously. This will limit any potential reactions that may happen because of inaccurate use.

Red light treatment works from the back to front to improve mitochondrial work in cells. This, thus, prompts a few skin benefits. Red light can enable the body to diminish skin inflammation, smooth skin tone, fix sun harm, blur scars and stretch imprints; it can even form collagen in the skin, which can lessen wrinkles and help mend wounds. Red light likewise decidedly impacts the lymphatic framework by expanding blood flow and in this way improving your body's capacity to detoxify.

Key Benefits:

- Upgraded blood dissemination
- Hostile to inflammatory impacts
- Expanded muscle recuperation
- Expanded collagen creation
- Brilliant skin
- Diminishes scars, wrinkles, and fine lines
- Rates wound recuperating
- Improved ripeness
- Expanded testosterone
- Diminishes torment

Why specifically utilize 630nm, 660nm, and 850nm wavelengths?

Different research ventures advance the benefits of various wavelengths for the treatment of specific conditions. It is commonly concurred that wavelengths somewhere in the range of 625nm and 900nm are the best for mending wounds and other skin conditions. At the lower end, 630nm and 660nm have all the earmarks of being favored. At longer wavelengths, 850nm and 880nm are the most beneficial.

A University of Chicago study found that the normal wavelength of cell tissue in the human body goes somewhere in the range of 600nm and 720nm, with 660nm being the mid-point. 660nm works superior to some other recurrence since it is nearer to the resounding recurrence of cell tissue, enabling it to assimilate better in hemoglobin. This is a red protein answerable for shipping oxygen in our blood. Your mitochondria can assimilate red light effectively at the 630nm and 660nm wavelengths, which generally match with the ingestion pinnacles of cytochrome c oxidase (the objective of light treatment).

The mitochondria's metabolic capacity is generally confined by a naturally dynamic particle called nitric oxide, which ties to cytochrome c oxidase and keeps it from utilizing oxygen. Red light withdraws this particle, permitting cytochrome c oxidase to continue its vitality delivering metabolic capacity.

Use throbbing or unfaltering light for more profound mending and relief from discomfort

It has been found that when LED lights are beat, body tissue can mend all the more quickly. At the point when it is given a ceaseless burst, it steadies the cell and eases the agony. At the point when a solitary recurrence beat light hits the cell, it invigorates the cell to begin delivering more protein than it regularly does, subsequently, the phone recuperates quicker. In any event, when the LED light source is removed, the cell proceeds with its recuperating. Rather than the beating light that is best for recuperating, a ceaseless, relentless light shaft can expel/dull agony, lessen inflammation and permits muscle tissue to unwind.

Keen on getting a light treatment gadget for home use? The NEW TrueLight™ Energy Square conveys patent-pending ideal Near Infrared, Deep Red, Red, and Yellow/Amber wavelengths with consistent or beating modes. TrueLight's interesting mix of wavelengths can respond with cell mitochondria to expand adenosine triphosphate (ATP) creation. Thus, expanded ATP generation can prompt quicker creation of collagen, vascular structures, DNA, RNA and different materials that are fundamental to your body's recuperating procedure. These wavelengths may improve blood course, lessen wrinkles and fine lines, increment muscle recuperation, decline torment and diminish joint inflammation just as skin redness/aggravation.

Advantages of Red Light Therapy

Photobiomodulation (light) treatment is a quickly developing innovation used to treat a large number of conditions that require incitement of mending, alleviation of agony and aggravation, and rebuilding of capacity.

Red and close to infrared light treatment has been clinically demonstrated to:

1. Fix harm from the sun and diminish your wrinkles

2. Speed muscle recuperation and upgrade top execution

3. Mend skin break out and imperfections

4. Blur scars and stretch imprints

5. Quicker twisted recuperating

6. Lessen joint aggravation

7. Lift testosterone levels

8. Help recuperation from Hypothyroidism

9. Upgrade collagen amalgamation and fix

10. Reestablish mitochondrial oxidation and vitality creation

Shockingly, not at all like numerous different medications used to address comparable conditions, there are for all intents and purposes no revealed symptoms. Serious overdosing of red/close infra-red light treatment could cause cerebral pains and fatigue. Note MitoGen entire body units and boards just utilize red and close infra-red light and don't radiate any UV light so there is zero chance of burn from the sun or DNA harm.

Red light can help with tooth affectability just as cleanliness. The tooth is made out of three layers. From back to front, there is the mash, the dentin, and the veneer. The deepest layer contains the veins and nerves and needs different layers to keep it secured. The dentin is the layer that encounters affectability when the lacquer is stripped away. At that point, the lacquer is the hard, defensive layer that watches within the tooth right down into the gums. Clearly, it is imperative to ensure the polish yet there are factors that debilitate this barrier and cause it to strip away.

Since the dentin layer is answerable for any affectability one may understanding, it is significant that this layer remains ensured and unblemished in order to not make any further harm the focal point of the tooth. Fortunately, the dentin is really ready to reestablish itself (dentinogenesis). Red light is said to accelerate this procedure. By focusing on and improving the digestion, red light can make the recovery increasingly successful and reduce the potential for affectability.

Tooth affectability is a typical tribulation among individuals that incredibly impacts one's everyday life. In this way, the way that red light treatment represents an answer is a major wellspring of expectation and energy in the dental world.

Red light treatment is a more current type of innovation that is being investigated in the dental consideration field. All things considered, it has advanced under the control of dental workplaces around the nation just as at home frameworks like Snow's teeth brightening unit. The advantages of red light treatment are really progressive and could change the round of oral wellbeing.

Medical advantages and Science of Red Light Therapy

Joint Health and Pain Managem

Red light treatment is presently being utilized to treat joint pain side effects on account of its capacity of animating collagen creation and revamping ligament. A 2009 Cochrane survey of red light treatment for rheumatoid joint inflammation reasoned that "Red light could be considered for momentary treatment for help of agony and morning solidness for RA patients, especially since it has scarcely any symptoms."

Indeed, even in the individuals who don't experience the ill effects of joint inflammation however have different indications of tissue harm or degeneration because of maturing, red light can in any case be advantageous. A recent report distributed in The Lancet appeared, "Red light lessens torment following treatment in intense neck torment and as long as 22 weeks after finishing of treatment in patients with ceaseless neck torment." Other investigations have discovered that in any event, when patients with musculoskeletal issue don't encounter less agony from red light treatment medicines, they have a high possibility of encountering "fundamentally improved practical results, for example, better scope of movement.

Cell restoration and expanded blood stream because of red light treatment are two key parts of improving joint and tissue wellbeing. Diminishing oxidative harm, which savages joints, and tweaking irritation are different ways that red light advantages delicate/connective tissue.

One utilization of red light treatment that is developing in ubiquity is switching indications of maturing on the skin (i.e, wrinkles and scarce differences). Results from a recent report distributed in Photomedicine and Laser Surgery showed both adequacy and wellbeing for red light treatment in advancing enemy of maturing skin restoration and intradermal collagen increment when looked at against controls. Scientists inferred that red infrared treatment "gives a safe, non-ablative, non-warm, atraumatic photobiomodulation treatment of skin tissue with high patient fulfillment rates."

Subjects treated with red light treatment experienced fundamentally improved skin composition, improved skin tone, improved surface/feeling, decreased skin unpleasantness, diminished indications of wrinkles and almost negligible differences, and expanded collagen thickness as estimated through ultrasonographic tests. Patients with rosacea and redness have likewise discovered help utilizing red light, even the individuals who can't endure higher-heat laser treatments.

Fix Of Muscle Tissue and Skin Rejuvenation

Red Light has been seen as helpful for advancing injury mending, tissue fix and skin revival, despite the fact that it does this through an alternate system of activity contrasted with numerous other laser reemerging medications. Red light treatment legitimately animates regenerative procedures in the skin through expanded cell multiplication, relocation and grip. Red light treatment has been appeared to emphatically influence skin cells through recovery of fibroblasts, keratinocytes and adjustment of invulnerable cells (counting pole cells, neutrophils and macrophages) all found inside skin tissue.

Resistance and Reduced Side Effects of Cancer Treatments

Research done by NASA related to the University of Alabama at Birmingham Hospital has indicated that red light innovation can effectively lessen manifestations experienced by malignant growth patients, including excruciating reactions caused from radiation or chemotherapy. Utilizing far red/close infrared light-emanating diode gadgets has been appeared to discharge long wavelength vitality as photons that animate cells to help in recuperating.

NASA tried whether red light could treat oral mucositis in malignancy patients, an exceptionally normal and excruciating symptom of chemotherapy and radiation, and inferred that 96 percent of patients experienced improvement in torment because of the red light treatment. Patients got the light treatment by a medical caretaker holding the WARP 75 gadget, which is generally the size of a grown-up human hand. The WARP gadget was held near the patient's face and neck for just 88 seconds every day for 14 days. Analysts expressed, "The red light gadget was very much endured with no unfavorable effects to bone marrow and foundational microorganism transplant patients... .The red light gadget can give a financially savvy treatment since the gadget itself is more affordable than one day at the clinic."

Comparable red light innovation is likewise now being

used for the treatment of pediatric cerebrum tumors, slow-mending wounds or diseases, diabetic skin ulcers, and genuine consumes.

Diminished Depression and Fatigue

Another approach to clarify the advantages of red light is through the perspective of Eastern medication. Light treatment improves wellbeing, invulnerability and recuperation, and can be contrasted with needle therapy's instrument of activity:

Light is a type of vitality, and our bodies are simply large vitality frameworks. Light has the ability to invigorate explicit meridian focuses and chakra zones in the human body.

Red is said to invigorate the first chakra in light of the fact that it relates most firmly with our endurance sense (henceforth why it gives us vitality and makes us act rapidly, so as to spur us to seek after things like cash, nourishment, sex, control, and so forth.).

While needle therapy utilizes small needles to accomplish substantial congruity by animating certain focuses in the body's vitality framework, light treatment utilizes engaged, unmistakable, red wavelengths similarly.

Red light has been demonstrated to be normally invigorating and related with improved states of mind by expanding fearlessness, energy, bliss, chuckling, care, mindfulness, and tactile incitement. While results fluctuate from patient to quiet, there's motivation to accept that red light has mental and enthusiastic advantages notwithstanding physical advantages.

Dr. Robert Calderhead, DrMedSci, FRSM, medicinal consultant to Photo therapeutics states "When viable wavelengths are gone for the photobiomodulation zone, destroy cells remain and safe, yet they get a jolt of energy from the immediate, a warm trade of vitality among photons and cell segments. This can help fix harmed cells. The 640nm is the most generally utilized wavelength for skin restoration."

Dr. Mary Dyson at Guy's Hospital in London, England indicated that "red light collagen lights at 633nm expanded the amalgamation of fibroblast development factor from macrophage cells."

Mount Sinai School of Medicine in New York City joined blue and red light treatment with collagen lights with Microdermabrasion on 22 subjects with gentle to serious facial skin inflammation vulgaris. Subjects were given eight (8) twenty (20) minute sessions, two times every week, switching back and forth among blue and red light with collagen lights, subjects were likewise given microdermabrasion before every session. The sore tally was decreased by 46% at four a month, and by 81% at twelve (12) weeks.

Dr. Mitchell Chasin, Medical Director of Reflections Center for Skin and Body in Livingston, New Jersey states "with LED you will see a decline in postoperative redness."

Dr. Mitchell Goldman, clinical educator of dermatology at the University of California San Diego and therapeutic chief at La Jolla Spa MD, La Jolla, CA states "Drove medications function admirably after any methodology that causes erythema (redness) and aggravation, including concoction strips, lasers and IPL.

Dr. Tina Alster of the Washington Institute of Dermatologic Laser Surgery, Washington DC, states " LED medications utilized with Fraxel laser, show a decrease in mending time of as much as half." Thirteen (13) subjects with scarcely discernible differences, wrinkles and photodamage, got nine (9) brief medicines over a five (5) week term. Sun harm at six a month and a half the dominant part showed a 25-half improvement at twelve (12) weeks: 91% revealed upgraded smoothness. Photobiology, April 2007

Seventy-six (76) subjects were isolated into four (4) gatherings. Medications were allowed two times every week for four a month. Scientists estimated the skin for versatility and melanin during the treatment time frame and for three (3) months following the medicines. Results demonstrated a noteworthy decrease of wrinkles (most extreme 36%) and an expansion of skin flexibility (greatest 19%). There was a checked increment in the measure of collagen and elastin filaments with exceptionally enacted fibroblast cells.

Dr. Harry T. Whelan, Professor of Neurology, Pediatrics and Hyperbaric Medicine at the Medical College of Wisconsin, found that diabetic skin ulcers and different injuries recuperated a lot quicker when presented to LEDs. Lab look into has indicated that the LEDs likewise develop human muscle and skin cells up to five (5) times quicker than typical. The examination, subsidized by NASA will look at the consequences for diabetic skin ulcers, genuine consumes and tissue wounds brought about by radiation and chemotherapy medicines. Dr. Whelan additionally expresses "The close infrared light discharged by these LEDs is by all accounts ideal for expanding vitality inside cells. LEDs support vitality to the cells and quicken recuperating.

Aces of red light treatment

– It can treat joint firmness and rheumatoid joint pain

joint inflammation

On the off chance that you are influenced with joint solidness or rheumatoid joint pain, red light treatment is perhaps the best alternative accessible out there to consider. That is on the grounds that the firm joints are in a situation to react flawlessly well to warm. Truth be told, you can utilize red light treatment to show signs of improvement results to defeat solid joints as opposed to warming cushions. That is on the grounds that the warmth created by red light treatment won't chill off rapidly. In this manner, you will have the option to get reliable outcomes alongside time.

Red light treatment can likewise warm up the joint reaction and inside tissues. In this way, you will have the option to get compelling outcomes without encountering surface warmth. At the point when you experience red light treatment, you will have the option to make your joints increasingly portable and usable. In this way, you can successfully fend off the hardening from getting more terrible. In the event that you can make it a propensity to expose your joints to red light treatment all the time, you will have the option to build the versatility of them by around 30%.

It has additionally been recognized that red light treatment can adequately upgrade the creation of collagen inside your body. Thus, you can modify collagen. This can lead you to diminishing the agony that you experience. It doesn't lead you to any symptoms when contrasted with the recommended drugs accessible to treat a similar wellbeing condition.

– It can improve the dissemination of blood

With the assistance of red light treatment, you can without much of a stretch improve the flow of blood too. At the end of the day, it can assist you with enhancing the manner in which how veins are functioning inside your body. At the point when the veins are working great, you can without much of a stretch enable blood to experience the body. In this way, you can conquer a wide range of vascular diseases that you will go over, for example, thickening of blood.

– It can assist you with recovering from wounds rapidly

On the off chance that you have any injuries in the body, you can get the assistance of red light treatment to recoup rapidly. This is one of the most unmistakable aces related with red light treatment. Your body has the regular capacity to mend alone. Be that as it may, the mending procedure would be quickened by invigorating the platelets. Then again, the lymphatic framework will be in a situation to gather squander items productively and expel them from your body.

The capacity to recoup from wounds is additionally upheld with an improved dissemination of blood. That is on the grounds that you can lessen growing and limit the odds of winding up with a contamination. In addition, red light treatment can assist you with reducing the odds of winding up with scars in the wake of mending.

The vast majority of the dermatologists out there on the planet want to utilize red light treatment to treat the individuals with recuperating wounds in view of the astonishing medical advantages that it can offer. The dermatologists additionally will in general utilize red light treatment to address skin restoration, wrinkles, skin joins and consume to mend. The dental specialists will in general utilize red light treatment to assist you with beating mouth blisters and mouth injuries, which occur around the mouth.

– It can support your invulnerability

The capacity of red light treatment to help your invulnerability is noteworthy. On the off chance that you need to diminish your odds of getting into sicknesses, this is probably the best choice accessible out there to consider. The capacity to improve your invulnerability will be offered through boosting the course of blood.

You will be intrigued to perceive how you are less inclined to wind up with normal wellbeing conditions, for example, cold and influenza. Then again, you can likewise get incredible help with limiting the odds of getting basic sicknesses.

– It can assist you with overcoming thyroid hormone related issues

Thyroid hormones assume a significant job in the general usefulness of your body. As it were, it is liable for helping you to keep up vitality levels and direct digestion. Be that as it may, an extensive level of the total populace is influenced by thyroid hormone related issues. Inside the United States, more than 20 million people are influenced by it.

At the point when you open your body to red light treatment, you can build the characteristic capacity of your body to help the usefulness of the thyroid organ. In this manner, your thyroid organ won't be influenced by your resistant framework.

– It can assist you with reducing torments

Individuals who subject themselves to red light treatment have better odds of beating the torments that they experience. This is another side-advantage that you can get with improved blood dissemination.

Regardless of whether you are influenced by torment related with joint inflammation or irritation, you can get exceptional outcomes with red light treatment. Thusly, you are emphatically urged to proceed with it and get the exceptional outcomes that please your direction.

– It can assist you with reducing muscle fits and eager legs muscles fits

Muscle issues or fits, alongside eager legs can be very baffling. They can even occupy you from completing your work every day. You won't have the option to get a decent rest around evening time as a result of this wellbeing condition. The principle explanation for muscle fits and eager legs is a decreased progression of blood. Accordingly, you have to consider improving the course of blood inside the body. That is the place red-light treatment can profit you with. At that point you can ensure that enough oxygen is shipped inside your body and you have a superior opportunity to defeat muscle fits and fretful legs.

With the assistance of red light treatment, you can improve the progression of blood. Alongside that, you will likewise have the option to improve the capacity that your muscles need to loosen up Your muscles won't be contracted a lot with red light treatment. On the off chance that you can make it a propensity to experience red light treatment all the time, you can totally defeat getting muscle fits. You will become hopelessly enamored with the enduring outcomes that are offered to you.

– It can profit your hair and skin

Any individual who is influenced with indications of untimely maturing will have the option to evaluate red light treatment and get positive outcomes. Truth be told, red light treatment is being utilized for an assortment of corrective purposes. You will have the option to diminish the presence of wrinkles just as every other indication of maturing in a viable way. Then again, you can remedially treat wounds, scars, and loss of hair with red light treatment. It can likewise assist you with overcoming rosacea skin issues and extreme skin inflammation.

At the point when you experience red light treatment, you can without much of a stretch lift the creation of collagen in the skin. This can profit your skin, hair and nails. Also, you will be driven towards showing signs of improvement skin appearance. You can get these outcomes with decreased scales on your skin, and lesser number of wrinkles. In addition, all individuals who experience red light treatment can invigorate the hair follicles to grow quicker.

– It can contribute towards your vitality levels and mind-set

Any individual who is anticipating improving the vitality levels and the state of mind will have the option to consider following red light treatment. You will have the option to upgrade vitality in cell levels. Hence, you can viably wind up with extraordinary outcomes. The effect that red light treatment can make on your thyroid hormone creation can likewise assist you with receiving exceptional outcomes.

In the event that you need to appreciate a superior mind-set, red light treatment is a decent choice to consider. You can without much of a stretch increment mental certainty and mental clearness with the help that you escape red light treatment. It can likewise assist you with enhancing general inspiration. With that, you can decrease uneasiness and ensure that you experience a quiet perspective consistently.

Precautions to red light therapy

Security measures

The significant contraindications for the utilization of light treatment are sicknesses that include the retina of the eye, (for example, diabetes) and the utilization of photosensitizing drugs (for example lithium, melatonin, phenothiazine antipsychotics and certain anti-infection agents). Individuals with a background marked by skin malignant growth and foundational lupus erythematosus ought to likewise maintain a strategic distance from this sort of treatment.

Phototherapy requires exceptional specialized hardware and prepared staff. Full range bulbs can bring about burns from the sun if the light doesn't have a diffuser which sift through the bright beams. This is the motivation behind why lights utilized in present day light treatment sift through bright light significantly and are believed to be more secure.

When photodynamic treatment is sought after, physical risks, for example, non-ionizing radiation created by the light-emanating gadget and synthetic dangers, for example, unwanted presentation to photosensitizing specialists applied to patients must be considered for safe use by the medicinal services proficient.

Individual defensive gear for photodynamic treatment ought to incorporate eye and skin insurance from synthetic concoctions and non-ionizing radiation. Building and regulatory gear controls that are prescribed for safe use ought to be carefully pursued.

Light treatment may significantly diminish neurodegeneration in Alzheimer's infection

Satisfactory inclusion of skin must be considered, and fitting material ought to be utilized to counteract infiltration of photosensitizing operators. Henceforth there is a requirement for research facility coats or other appropriate apparel that can cover however much uncovered skin as could reasonably be expected, and furthermore hinder the approaching radiation.

Capacity of a texture to ensure against radiation is regularly estimated by the UV assurance factor (UPF), which demonstrates the amount of the powerful UV portion gets ingested to secure the skin. The rating is generally founded on the fiber thickness and structure, in spite of the fact that pre-treatment with an UV-restraining fixing is likewise a choice.

Symptoms of light treatment

Light treatment that includes just unmistakable light is commonly viewed as sheltered. All things considered, the utilization of phototherapy for individuals with medicate safe non-regular gloom can bring about a hyperactive state called craziness. In these uncommon cases light treatment must be decreased or halted and the condition satisfactorily treated.

Any treatment where the patient is presented to bright radiation isn't totally without its dangers – including untimely maturing of the skin and an expanded plausibility for skin malignant growth improvement further down the road. Eye strain and impermanent cerebral pains brought about by the light are additionally regularly detailed, in spite of the fact that these side effects don't appear to demonstrate any lasting damage.

In photodynamic treatment, symptoms vary contingent on the sort of photosensitizer utilized, with methyl aminolevulinate tending to create the most extreme agony during treatment and possibly a higher possibility of ensuing hyperpigmentation. Patients now and again additionally experience a flare of skin break out that is short lived in nature.

Photosensitivity responses activated by light include redness, stinging and consuming and they for the most part die down three weeks after the treatment. Unfavorably susceptible responses, for example, hives and skin inflammation can show up at the region of contact inside a couple of hours after introduction to the cream.

Depending on unsubstantiated employments of light treatment while deferring or keeping away from ordinary treatment for disease can have desperate results. That is the motivation behind why a multidisciplinary approach must be sought after, and there is likewise a likelihood to pre-treat the tumor cells to make them increasingly defenseless to photodynamic treatment.

Safety measures Before Beginning Red Light Therapy

While red light treatment is broadly viewed as totally

sheltered, there are a couple of insurances.

The most widely recognized hazard related with this treatment is sparkling it in your eyes. Not unreasonably red or infrared light itself is harming to your eyes, however the gadgets can create high glare. Respectable items will accompany eye insurance, and it ought to be worn during each facial treatment. In the event that you are utilizing the light for non-facial applications, for example, wound consideration or help with discomfort, simply be mindful so as to not to sparkle the light in your eyes. (The equivalent goes for your pets.) Never look straightforwardly into the red light treatment gadget.

If it's not too much trouble read this extra rundown of precautionary measures and contra-signs gave by Thor Laser (a pioneer in restorative red and infrared light treatment or LLLT). It incorporates notes for alerts for:

- pregnancy
- malignant growth
- drain
- insusceptible suppressant drugs

A few investigations exhibit the advantages of low-control light treatment on wound recuperating.

Nonetheless, the utilization of LED as a helpful asset stays disputable. There are questions with respect to the equity or not of natural impacts advanced by LED and LASER. One target of this survey was to decide the natural impacts that help the utilization of LED on wound mending. Another goal was to recognize LED's parameters for the treatment of wounds. The organic impacts and parameters of LED will be contrasted with those of LASER. Writing was acquired from online databases, for example, Medline, PubMed, Science Direct and Scielo. The pursuit was confined to thinks about distributed in English and Portuguese from 1992 to 2012. Sixty-eight investigations in vitro and in creatures were examined. Driven and LASER advance comparable organic impacts, for example, decline of provocative cells, expanded fibroblast expansion, incitement of angiogenesis, granulation tissue arrangement and expanded combination of collagen. The light parameters are likewise comparative among LED and LASER. The organic impacts are subject to light parameters, chiefly wavelength and portion. This survey clarifies the significance of characterizing parameters for the utilization of light gadgets.

Red light treatment is a helpful method you have to attempt.

Red light treatment is an imaginative restorative procedure that utilizations red, low-level wavelengths to treat skin issues, similar to scars, wrinkles, tireless injuries, and different conditions. In its fundamental structure, red light treatment works by creating a biochemical impact in the cells that fortifies the mitochondria, which are the powerhouses of the cell and where cell vitality is made.

Red Light Therapy in Black Mountain, North Carolina

At Greenspan Wellness Center, we are the main spot operating at a profit Mountain, North Carolina region to offer red light treatment, and we gladly offer this administration as a feature of our full lineup of choices. Before prescribing red light treatment, we will cautiously break down your condition and decide whether this treatment alternative is directly for your before pushing ahead with treatment.

One of the fundamental advantages of red light treatment is that it is sheltered and effortless with no significant symptoms. In the event that you have an inclination that you have attempted several meds, both over the counter and remedy, and numerous other conventional arrangements, red light treatment might be the appropriate response you are searching for to discover changeless alleviation. Our group consistently pursues all vital security precautionary measures during every red light treatment session to guarantee the procedure is totally sheltered and that you experience the most advantage conceivable.

We would be glad to disclose to you increasingly about red light treatment, how it works, and how it can profit numerous wellbeing conditions. Get in touch with us at Greenspan Wellness Center today to discover more and to set up your underlying interview.

Conceivable Side Effects of Red Light Therapy

The National Center for Biotechnology Information has noticed, "The non-obtrusive nature and practically complete nonattendance of symptoms empower further testing in dermatology." While there isn't sufficient data thought about the impacts of red light on the eyes, it is a smart thought to utilize precautionary measure and consistently wear defensive eyewear.

How Do You Get Red Light Therapy?

On the off chance that you are keen on accepting red light treatment medicines, you should initially counsel your dermatologist, oncologist, orthopedic, essential consideration specialist, rheumatologist or nervous system specialist about treatment alternatives. To locate a neighborhood red light treatment choice, numerous spas, restorative offices, and wellness studios offer different types of red light treatment. From little wands to whole beds, there are additionally various FDA endorsed at-home gadgets currently being sold coming up and on the web. You can look at the best at home red light treatment gadgets here.

Going Ahead with Red Light Therapy

We are continually getting developing proof from clinical research and concentrates supporting the medical advantages of red and NIR light treatment. From improved psychological execution to help with discomfort, red light treatment has legitimately earned its ongoing prominence.

The Effects of Red Light on Bio Organisms

Research underpins that particular light wavelengths

cause a biochemical impact in cells that lift the vitality creation of mitochondria. An investigation in the diary Seminars in Cutaneous Medicine and Surgery notes, mitochondria in the skin cells can assimilate these light particles, boosting a cell's vitality with the formation of adenosine triphosphate (ATP). 2

You can think about the mitochondria as the powerhouse of the cell. By expanding ATP creation, the cell has more vitality to work all the more proficiently and fix harm.

Driven light treatment is additionally thought to add to working up the cell's cancer prevention agent and mitigating safeguard frameworks.

At the point when red light treatment is utilized with drugs, for example, lithium, melatonin, phenothiazine antipsychotics and certain anti-microbials, it's alluded to as photodynamic treatment. In this kind of treatment, light is just utilized as an enacting specialist.

Red Light Therapy versus Prescriptions

Irritation is commonly treated with meds, which can have genuine reactions. The utilization of red light treatment in treating irritation without the symptoms of conventional meds is demonstrating incredible guarantee.

NSAIDs

Over the counter assortments of NSAIDs (non-steroidal mitigating drugs) incorporate headache medicine, ibuprofen (Advil), and naproxen (Aleve). As indicated by the Cleveland Clinic, normal symptoms of NSAIDs include:

Stomach agony and indigestion

Stomach ulcers

An inclination to drain more, particularly when taking headache medicine. Your primary care physician may instruct you to quit taking NSAIDs before medical procedure. Ask your PCP before taking NSAIDs in the event that you are on blood-diminishing meds, (for example, Coumadin).

Cerebral pains and unsteadiness

Ringing in the ears

Unfavorably susceptible responses, for example, rashes, wheezing, and throat growing

Liver or kidney issues. On the off chance that you have any kidney issues, you shouldn't take NSAIDs without checking with your primary care physician.

- Hypertension
- Leg growing
- Gas
- Feeling enlarged
- Queasiness
- Retching
- The runs or potentially stoppage 3

Enlarged from Steroid Use

Steroids

The utilization of steroids is regularly a treatment for battling irritation. Steroids decline irritation and smother the safe framework, which is useful when it begins assaulting sound tissue.

Be that as it may, long haul utilization of steroids can prompt vision issues, hypertension, and osteoporosis. While endorsing steroids, your PCP will gauge the advantages and dangers with you.

Enhancements

A few enhancements have demonstrated guarantee in treating aggravation, including fish oil, lipoic corrosive, and curcumin. A few flavors are additionally noted for assuaging irritation, including ginger, garlic, turmeric, and cayenne.

Viability and Safety of Red Light Therapy

Red light treatment doesn't make harm the skin's surface, which contrasts from laser or exceptional beat light (IPL) treatment. Light wavelengths work by making harm the external layer of skin, instigating tissue fix. In an unexpected way, red light enters just around 5 millimeters into the skin, legitimately animating cell recovery and collagen generation.

Full-range light can bring about burns from the sun if the light doesn't have a diffuser which sift through the bright wavelengths. Lights utilized in present day light treatment that channel out bright beams are viewed as more secure, yet alert ought to be utilized for photodynamic treatment.

As noted in News-Medical.net, "When photodynamic treatment is sought after, physical risks, for example, non-ionizing radiation delivered by the light-producing gadget and substance perils, for example, unwanted presentation to photosensitizing specialists applied to patients must be considered for safe use by the medicinal services proficient." 4

How Red Light Therapy Works for Cancer Treatment

In an investigation looking at the impacts of red light treatment on tumor development, it was discovered that medicines gave some guarantee without displaying security concerns. 5

"The present examination neglected to show a hurtful impact of entire body red light on tumor development in a trial model of UV-incited SCC. There was a transient and little decrease in relative tumor territory in the treatment bunch contrasted and controls. This investigation recommends that LLLT ought not be retained from disease patients on an empiric premise."

Treatment of Skin Conditions

A recent report inspected the wellbeing of red light treatment in treating various skin conditions that require a decrease of aggravation while concentrating the security of the medicines. The specialists finished up:

"In pigmentary clutters, for example, vitiligo, LLLT can expand pigmentation by animating melanocyte expansion and diminish depigmentation by hindering autoimmunity. Fiery illnesses, for example, psoriasis and skin inflammation can likewise profit. The non-obtrusive nature and practically complete nonattendance of symptoms empowers further testing in dermatology."

Are There Medical Conditions Tied to Red Light Therapy?

There are no investigations attached straightforwardly to the utilization of red light treatment and the individuals who experience photosensitivity responses, it is prescribed that you do a skin affectability test before experiencing any light treatment. 6

People respond contrastingly to introduction to light. While most have no response, some may create unreasonable redness or aggravation. In the event that you notice any redness, disturbance, irritation, or different responses, it is recommended that you contact the gadget maker and counsel with your social insurance proficient.

Regularly any redness or disturbance will vanish inside a couple of hours or days. In any case, any difficult response that doesn't vanish in this time ought to be accounted for to your primary care physician.

On the off chance that you are taking any meds, it is prescribed that you counsel with your primary care physician before starting any new light routine to guarantee there won't be antagonistic responses. Certain anti-infection agents and prescriptions make you additional touchy to light.

Fundamental Safety for Red Light Treatments

With any wellspring of light, gazing straightforwardly at the bulbs may cause eye strain that can instigate cerebral pains, headaches, or sickness. Glare from LED bulbs may likewise cause distress. In any setting where light treatment is being managed, it is prescribed to wear defensive eyewear.

Extra Benefits of Red Light Therapy

The safe and insignificantly intrusive nature of red light treatment is proceeding to be examined. Healthline takes note of the promising advantages of red light and NIR light medicines:

- advances wound recuperating and tissue fix
- improves hair development in individuals with androgenic alopecia
- help for the momentary treatment of carpal passage disorder
- animates mending of moderate recuperating wounds, similar to diabetic foot ulcers
- lessens psoriasis sores
- helps with momentary alleviation of torment and morning solidness in individuals with rheumatoid joint pain
- decreases a portion of the reactions of disease medications, including oral mucositis
- improves skin appearance and fabricates collagen to lessen wrinkles and barely recognizable differences
- retouches sun harm
- keeps repeating mouth blisters from herpes simplex infection contaminations
- improves the strength of joints in individuals with degenerative osteoarthritis of the knee
- lessens scars

- eases agony and aggravation in individuals with torment in the Achilles' ligaments 7

Side effects of red light therapy

5 Benefits of Red Light Therapy

1. Expanded Immunity and Reduced Side Effects of Cancer Treatments

Research done by NASA related to the University of Alabama at Birmingham Hospital has demonstrated that red light innovation can effectively decrease side effects experienced by malignant growth patients, including difficult reactions caused from radiation or chemotherapy. Utilizing far red/close infrared light-emanating diode gadgets (called High Emissivity Aluminiferous Luminescent Substrate, or HEALS for this situation) has been appeared to discharge long wavelength vitality as photons that invigorate cells to help in mending.

NASA tried whether HEALS could treat oral mucositis in malignant growth patients, an exceptionally normal and difficult symptom of chemotherapy and radiation, and reasoned that 96 percent of patients experienced improvement in torment because of the HEALS treatment. Patients got the light treatment by a medical caretaker holding the WARP 75 gadget, which is generally the size of a grown-up human hand. The WARP gadget was held near the patient's face and neck for just 88 seconds day by day for 14 days. Scientists expressed, "The HEALS gadget was very much endured with no antagonistic effects to bone marrow and immature microorganism transplant patients… .The HEALS gadget can give a practical treatment since the gadget itself is more affordable than one day at the emergency clinic." (6)

Comparative HEALS innovation is additionally now being used for the treatment of pediatric mind tumors, slow-mending wounds or diseases, diabetic skin ulcers, and genuine consumes.

2. Wound Healing and Tissue Repair

Light in the ghastly scope of 600 to 1,300 nanometers has been seen as helpful for advancing injury mending, tissue fix and skin restoration, despite the fact that it does this through an alternate system of activity contrasted with numerous other laser reemerging medicines. Most laser treatments utilized in dermatology workplaces utilize extraordinary beat light to advance skin revival by instigating optional tissue fix. At the end of the day, they influence purposeful harm to either the epidermis or the dermis of the skin so as to trigger irritation, trailed by recuperating.

Red light treatment really sidesteps this underlying dangerous advance and rather straightforwardly invigorates regenerative procedures in the skin through expanded cell multiplication, movement and grip. Red light treatment has been appeared to decidedly influence skin cells through recovery of fibroblasts, keratinocytes and adjustment of invulnerable cells (counting pole cells, neutrophils and macrophages) all found inside skin tissue.

3. Against Aging Effects for Skin and Hair Loss

One utilization of red light laser treatment that is developing in notoriety is turning around indications of maturing on the skin (i.e, wrinkles and almost negligible differences). Results from a recent report distributed in Photomedicine and Laser Surgery showed both viability and security for red light treatment in advancing enemy of maturing skin revival and intradermal collagen increment when thought about against controls. (7) Researchers inferred that red infrared treatment "gives a safe, non-ablative, non-warm, atraumatic photobiomodulation treatment of skin tissue with high patient fulfillment rates."

Subjects treated with red light treatment experienced altogether improved skin appearance, improved skin tone, improved surface/feeling, diminished skin unpleasantness, decreased indications of wrinkles and scarce differences, and expanded collagen thickness as estimated through ultrasonographic tests. Patients with rosaceaand redness have likewise discovered alleviation utilizing LLLT, even the individuals who can't endure higher-heat laser treatments.

One more enemy of maturing impact of red light treatment is switching male pattern baldness and invigorating follicle development, which works in a large number of indistinguishable ways from red light treatment for wound recuperating. Results have been blended by examines, however at any rate a moderate segment of both male and female patients have had positive outcomes for turning around hairlessness/male pattern baldness when utilizing LLLT. (8)

4. Improved Joint and Musculoskeletal Health

Red light treatment is presently being utilized to treat joint pain side effects because of its capacity of invigorating collagen generation and modifying ligament. A 2009 Cochrane survey of red light treatment for rheumatoid arthritisconcluded that "LLLT could be considered for transient treatment for alleviation of torment and morning solidness for RA patients, especially since it has scarcely any symptoms."

Indeed, even in the individuals who don't experience the ill effects of joint pain however have different indications of tissue harm or degeneration because of maturing, LLLT can in any case be useful. A recent report distributed in The Lancet appeared, "LLLT decreases torment following treatment in intense neck torment and as long as 22 weeks after finishing of treatment in patients with incessant neck torment." Other examinations have discovered that in any event, when patients with musculoskeletal issue don't encounter less torment from red light treatment medications, they have a high possibility of encountering "fundamentally improved utilitarian results, for example, better scope of movement.

Cell restoration and expanded blood stream because of red light treatment are two key parts of improving joint and tissue wellbeing. Diminishing oxidative harm, which ruffians joints, and regulating aggravation are different ways that LLLT benefits delicate/connective tissue.

5. Decreased Depression and Fatigue

Another approach to clarify the advantages of red light is through the viewpoint of Eastern medication. Ask a Traditional Chinese Medicine specialist how light improves wellbeing, insusceptibility and recuperation, and the individual in question will probably contrast it with needle therapy's component of activity:

Light is a type of vitality, and our bodies are simply large vitality frameworks. Light has the ability to invigorate explicit meridian focuses and chakrazones in the human body.

Red is said to invigorate the first chakra on the grounds that it connects most unequivocally with our endurance sense (subsequently why it gives us vitality and makes us act rapidly, so as to propel us to seek after things like cash, nourishment, sex, control, and so on.).

While needle therapy utilizes small needles to accomplish substantial agreement through invigorating certain focuses in the body's vitality framework, light treatment utilizes engaged, unmistakable, red wavelengths similarly.

Is there anything I can do to encounter red light treatment benefits quicker?

The exploration exhibited in "Green tea and red light: an amazing do in skin revival", asserts that putting green tea sacks on the skin for 20 minutes before treatment expands the counter maturing advantage by 10-crease. Outstandingly, results acknowledged in 10 months of light treatment happened in only multi month.

I took a stab at utilizing green tea packs all over before red light treatment. Be that as it may, I found the entire procedure just excessively muddled. In spite of the chaos, I like the exploration. In this way, I am going to utilize a green tea serum 20 minutes before light treatment. Presently, this doesn't copy the examination yet it can't hurt.

What are the reactions of red light treatment?

Essentially, none of the clinical preliminaries I looked into announced any genuine unfavorable impacts. Red LED light is viewed as sheltered to utilize. Red light treatment doesn't include introduction to bright (UV) radiation. When contrasted with different mediations, for example, retinoic corrosive, dermabrasion, concoction strips, and laser reemerging, there is no personal time. In fact, this is a non-ablative treatment without torment, redness, aggravation, stripping or danger of contamination.

The security profile is to such an extent that LED light treatment can be stacked with different medications. Consider skin needling, and microdermabrasion pursued by red light. Besides, almost certainly, consolidating medicines will have a synergistic impact with improved corrective results. Everything considered, this is only an incredible treatment to use at home.

Do I have to shield my eyes from red light?

A few investigations report that red light introduction might be helpful to the eye. Be that as it may, these are your eyes. Along these lines, except if guided by a doctor to open your eyes to red light, I would decide in favor of alert. In the event that you are uncovering your full face to LED red light, I propose covering the eyes with little eye goggles.

Are successful red light treatment benefits conceivable with the utilization of red light treatment at home?

Indeed, a non-therapeutic spa is probably going to offer red light treatment utilizing LED lights and not a laser. Indeed, this is frequently a similar unit you can buy for red light treatment at home. Obviously, a dermatologist will have the decision of LED lights or a powerful laser.

Yet, as per noted Harvard analyst, Michael Hamblin, a laser isn't required for powerful treatment and red light treatment at home is similarly as successful as an expert laser. Hamblin states, "The greater part of the early work in this field was done with different sorts of lasers, and it was imagined that laser light had some uncommon qualities not controlled by light from other light sources, for example, daylight, fluorescent or radiant lights and now LEDs. Notwithstanding, every one of the examinations contrasting lasers with equal light sources with comparable wavelength and power thickness of their outflow, have found basically no distinction between them."

What sort of LED light would it be a good idea for me to purchase to get most extreme red light treatment benefits?

The significance of wavelength or nanometers

The most detailed wavelength extend for red light

treatment in the clinical examinations I looked into was between 630-680 nm. When buying a red LED light, the producer or merchant ought to have the option to give the wavelength. On the off chance that they can't, at that point purchase from another person. Most importantly, it is imperative to concentrate on shading as far as wavelength or nm and not what shading the producer reports the unit as delivering. Red light happens with a wavelength between 620 to 700 nm.

The significance of light force or power

Notwithstanding nm, force or light power influences the term of treatment. More noteworthy power approaches a shorter treatment time. It is here that it gets truly befuddling. In the event that you are looking at items dependent on joules, ensure that joules are expressed in joules every second per square centimeter over a similar timeframe. This gives you a standard unit of measure since joules can be accounted for in various manners. On the off chance that you don't do this, you are contrasting one type with a totally different type. Another approach to think about the power between various units is to take a gander at mW(milliwatts)/cm2.

Studies show skin improvement with both hand-held

gadgets and huge LED boards. A hand-held unit that is put straightforwardly against the skin is commonly more viable than a light board. This is on the grounds that the closer the light source is to the skin the more noteworthy the light power.

You may find out about beat LED lights. Beating is a system used to limit heat harm delivered by lasers. Be that as it may, red LED light doesn't deliver heat. Along these lines, light beating isn't fundamental.

Now, on the off chance that it feels like you need a material science certificate to see this, well, you are not a long way from reality. Nonetheless, the quantity of clinical examinations that show proof of the adequacy of LED treatment in photorejuvenation utilizing an assortment of LED light sources with various power forces is consoling.

www.ingramcontent.com/pod-product-compliance
Lightning Source LLC
Chambersburg PA
CBHW031107250726
48655CB00004B/1609